A QUESTRON™ ELECTRONIC

MORE HOW, WHY, WHERE & WHEN

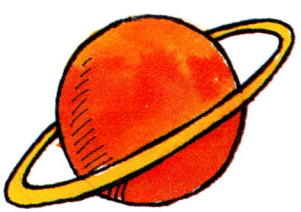
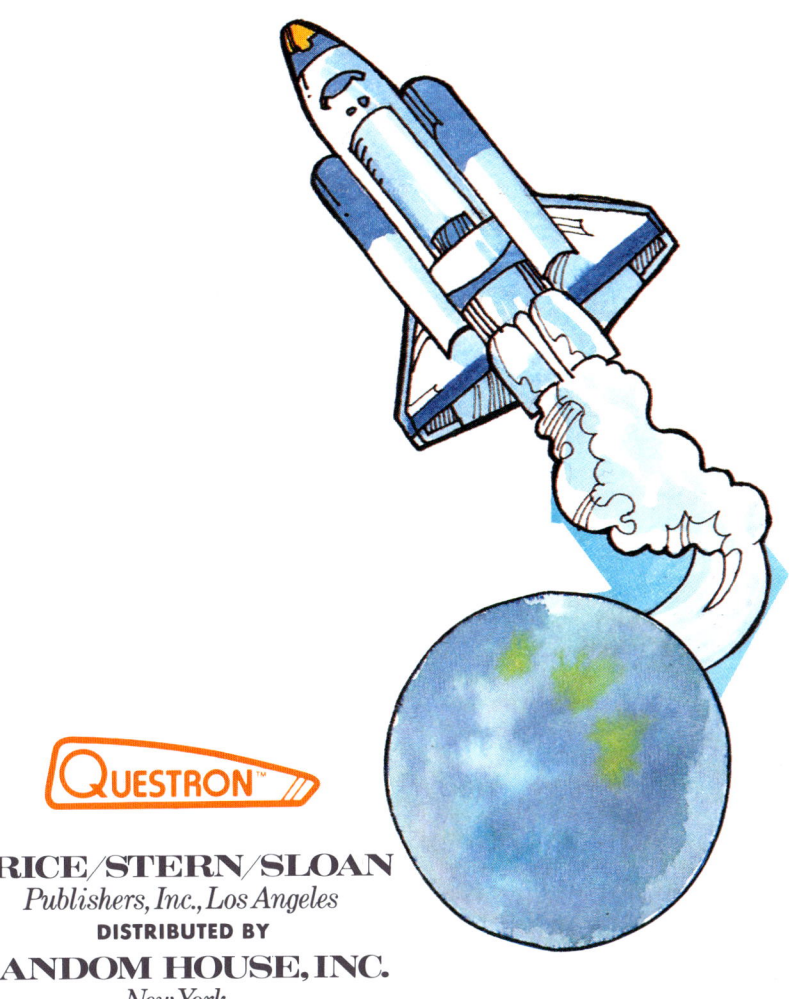

PRICE/STERN/SLOAN
Publishers, Inc., Los Angeles
DISTRIBUTED BY
RANDOM HOUSE, INC.
New York

THE QUESTRON™ SYSTEM
COMBINING FUN WITH LEARNING

This is one of a series of **QUESTRON ELECTRONIC BOOKS**. As part of **THE QUESTRON SYSTEM**, it provides a unique aid to learning.

Questron Electronic Books are available for all ages and will provide endless hours of challenging entertainment. Correct answers are determined immediately, and Questron Electronic Books can be used over and over.

QUESTRON itself is a unique electronic device that contains a magic microchip which "senses" correct or incorrect answers by signaling the user with a "right" or "wrong" sound, along with appropriate lights. In addition, it sometimes provides a "victory" sound and flashing light pattern when certain sets of questions or games are completed. QUESTRON, powered by a nine-volt battery, should have an especially long life, since it is activated only when an answer is being sought. The Questron Electronic Wand is on sale wherever Questron Electronic Books are sold and can be used with any book which is part of the Questron Electronic Book series.

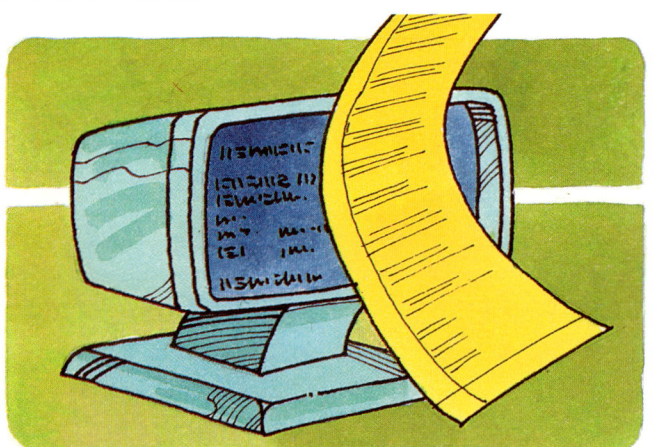

QUESTRON Project Director: Roger Burrows
Educational Consultant: Beverley Dietz
Writer: Yvette Lodge
Illustrator: Dave LaFleur
Graphic Designers: Judy Walker, Jamie Cain

Copyright © 1984 by Price/Stern/Sloan Publishers, Inc. All rights reserved under International and Pan-American Copyright Conventions. No part of this publication may be reproduced, stored in a retrieval system, or transmitted in any form or by any means, electronic, mechanical, photocopying, recording or otherwise, without the prior written permission of the publisher. Published by Price/Stern/Sloan Publishers, Inc., 410 North La Cienega Boulevard, Los Angeles, California 90048. Distributed by Random House, Inc., 201 East 50th Street, New York, New York 10022   ISBN: 0-394-87696-2
Manufactured in Hong Kong   1 2 3 4 5 6 7 8 9 0

QUESTRON is a trademark of Price/Stern/Sloan Publishers, Inc.

Patents Pending

QUESTRON

Hold **QUESTRON** <u>at this angle</u> and press the activator button firmly on the page.

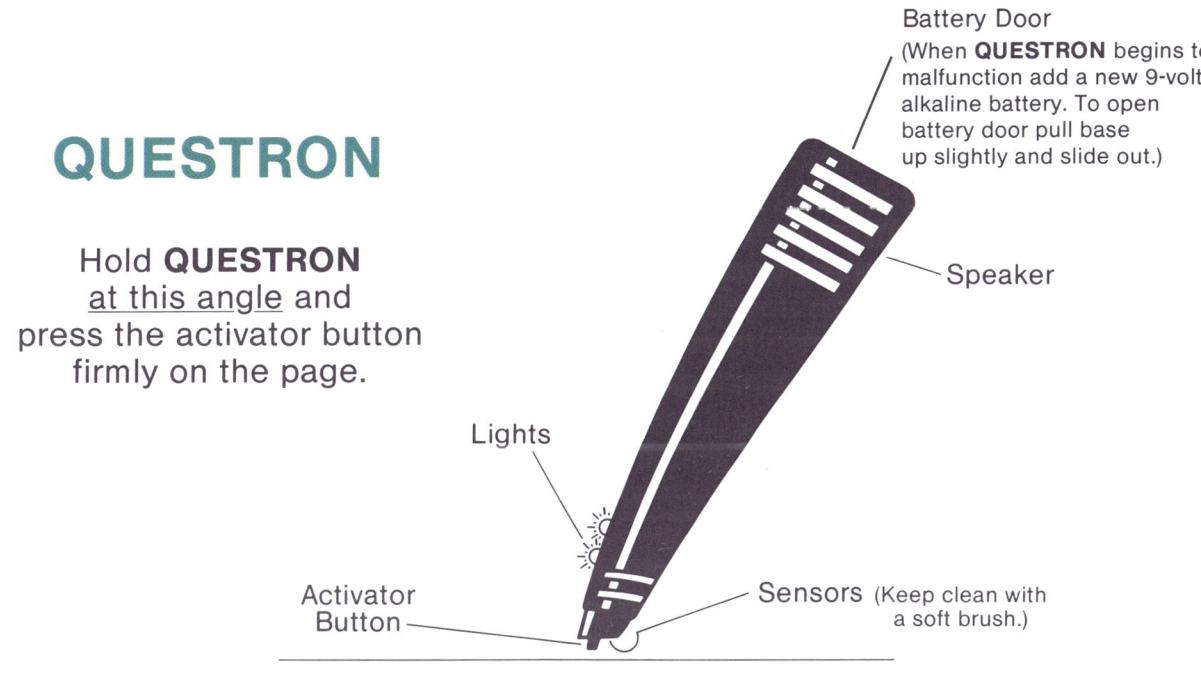

HOW TO USE QUESTRON

PRESS
Press **QUESTRON** firmly on the shape below, then lift it off.

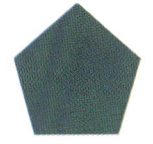

TRACK
Press **QUESTRON** down on "Start" and keep it pressed down as you move to "Finish."

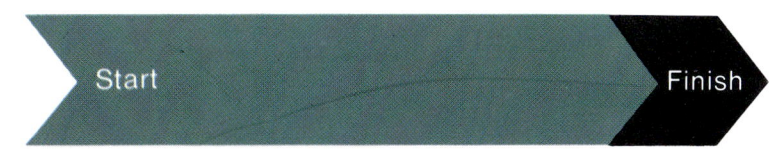

RIGHT & WRONG WITH QUESTRON

Press **QUESTRON** on the square.

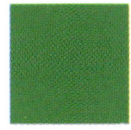

See the green light flash. Hear the sound. This green light and sound say "You are correct."

Press **QUESTRON** on the circle.

Hear the victory sound. Don't be dazzled by the flashing lights. You deserve them.

Press **QUESTRON** on the triangle.

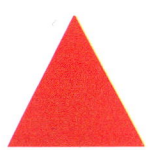

The red light and sound say "Try again." Lift **QUESTRON** off the page and wait for the sound to stop.

PICTURE THIS

Today's cameras look complex when compared to early cameras, but the principals of photography are still the same. A camera is a light-tight box with a hole covered by a shutter. The hole is called an aperture. Film, which has been chemically treated to be sensitive to light, is inside the camera. A button is pressed to open the shutter. Light, reflected off an object and focused through a lens, enters the camera and strikes the film.

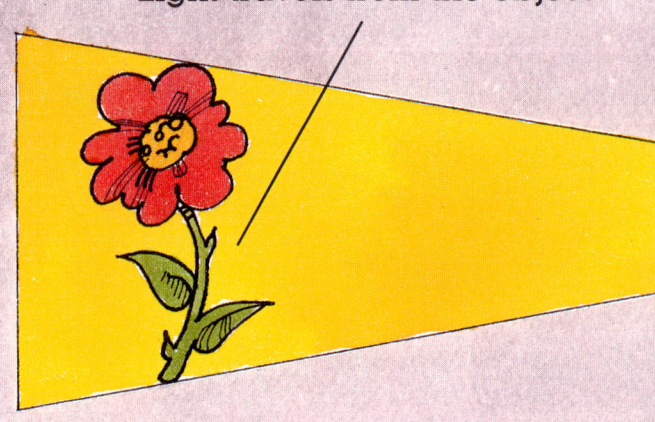

Light travels from the object

Read each question. Then press **QUESTRON** on the colored square next to the right answer.

The first photograph was taken by French scientist Joseph Nicéphore Niepce. It took eight hours to expose! When was it taken?

1903 1859
1826 1887

Doctors are able to take photographs of our internal organs and reproduce the images as shadow pictures. What are these pictures called?

Radio-grams   Cardio-graphs
X-rays   Litho-graphs

When you photograph an object, an image appears on the film. What does the image of the word "PICTURE" look like?

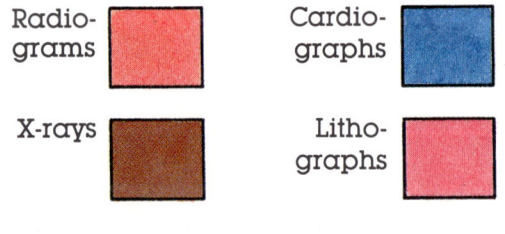

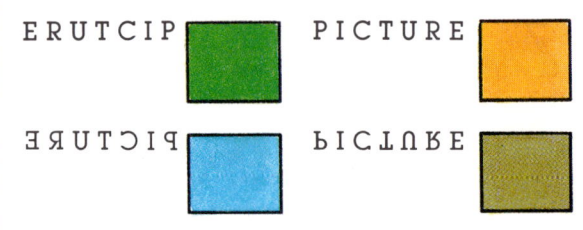

The origins of black and white film date back to 1787, when a German, Johann Schulze, placed stencils around glass bottles that contained a special mixture. When exposed to sunlight, the part of the mixture not covered by stencils turned black. The mixture contained two elements. One was silver nitrate. What was the other?

Chalk   Bromide
Gelatin   Crystal

Photographers often use a three-legged device to hold their cameras perfectly still. What is this device called?

An easel   A prop
A tripod   A boom

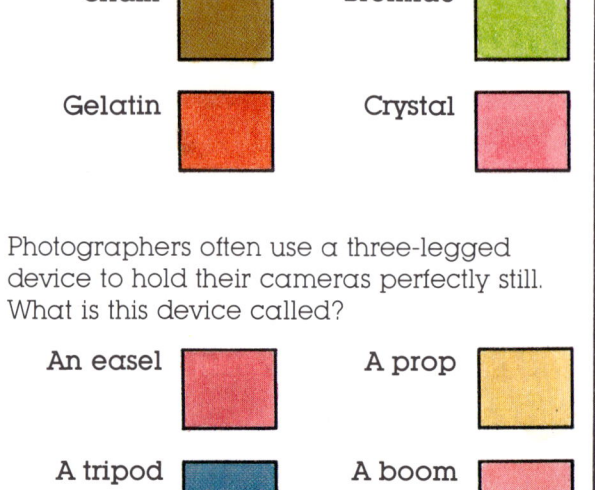

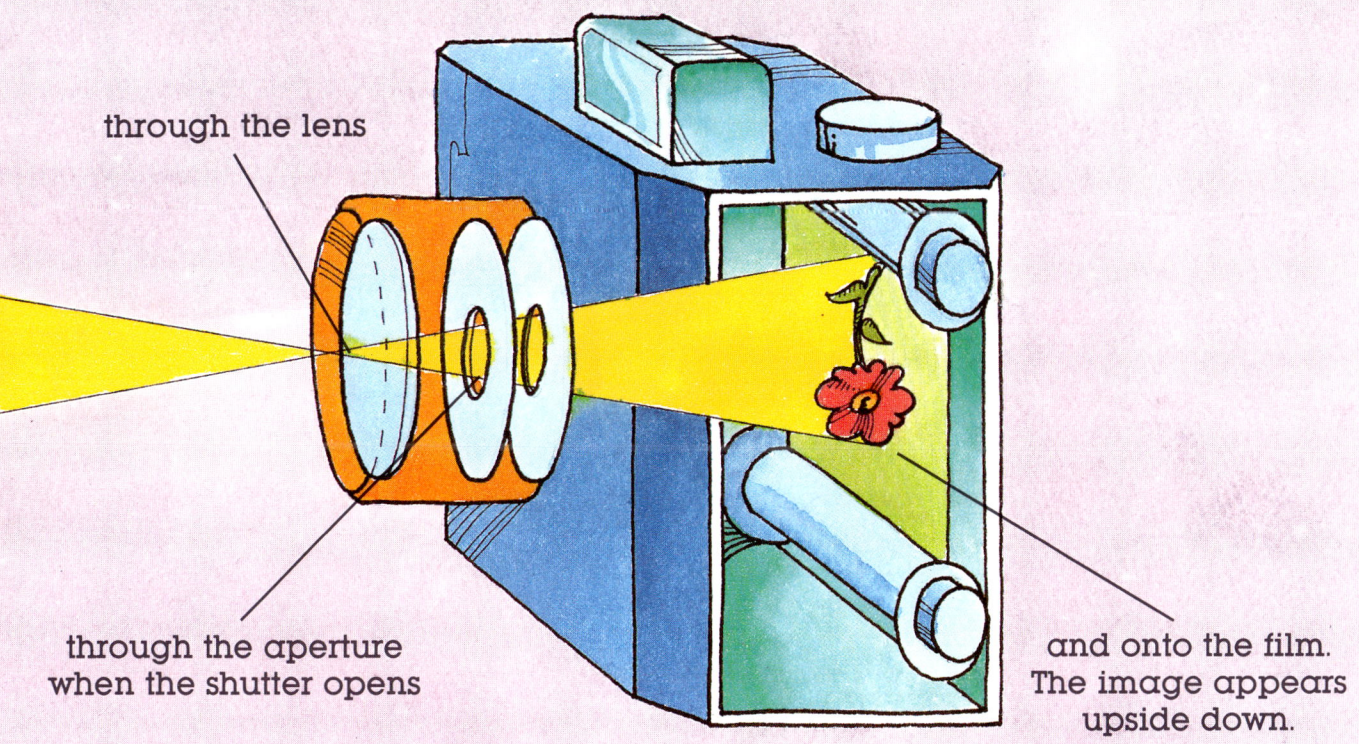

through the lens

through the aperture when the shutter opens

and onto the film. The image appears upside down.

Many people like to use Polaroid Land film cameras, which produce finished photographs in seconds. These photographs still have to be developed with chemicals. Where are the chemicals located?

In the camera   In each print

In the film container   In a camera attachment

The fastest cameras in the world are used by doctors and scientists. They help record information during surgery and in experiments. These cameras can take a picture in millionths of a second. How many millionths?

600   8

240   57

After perfecting the camera, people went on to develop motion pictures. The first "movies" open to the public were presented in New York in 1894. The audience was able to see 10 short films in one viewing. What do you think the admission price was?

Five dollars   Two dollars

10 cents   50 cents

Lenses are designed to sharpen and to reduce or enlarge images. The first known use of lenses was in the 13th century when a man used them to make a telescope. Who was he?

Galileo   Roger Bacon

Hans Lippershey   Leonardo da Vinci

COMMUNICATIONS

Until the age of technology, information was passed from person to person through speech or handwriting. Today we can use complex machinery that enables us to reach the farthest corners of the world within seconds.

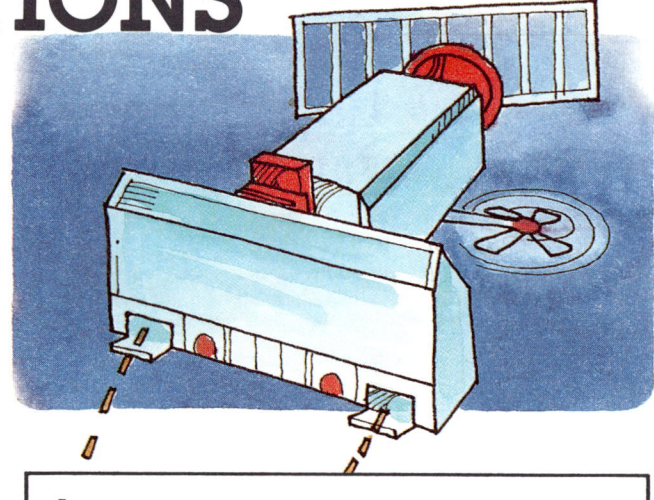

Read each question. Then press **QUESTRON** on the colored square next to the right answer.

Satellites

Television programs are often transmitted via man-make satellites that orbit the earth and beam signals from one continent to another. The first such satellite was launched in 1962. What was it called?

Pioneer	Luna
Explorer	Telstar

Broadcasting

When radio was first introduced, people disliked it for its lack of privacy. The first broadcast of a human voice amazed the world. When did it happen?

1860	1888
1906	1942

Language

There are about 490,000 words in today's English language. Most people use fewer than 5,000 in everyday speech. What is the most used word in spoken English?

A	I
The	And

Fiber Optics

Fiber optics are relatively new to the world of communications. Each optical fiber is as fine as a human hair and can transmit over 2,000 telephone messages at once. Calls are sent along the fibers by laser light pulses. What material is used to make optical fibers?

Plastic	Rubber
Wire	Glass

Telegraph Service

The first telegraph message was sent out in 1844. Letters were represented by long and short electrical impulses. The code is still widely used. Who invented it?

Samuel Morse	Alexander Graham Bell
William Caxton	Heinrich Hertz

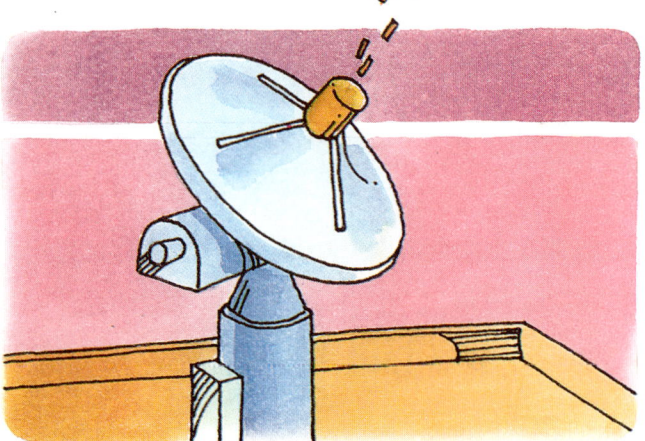

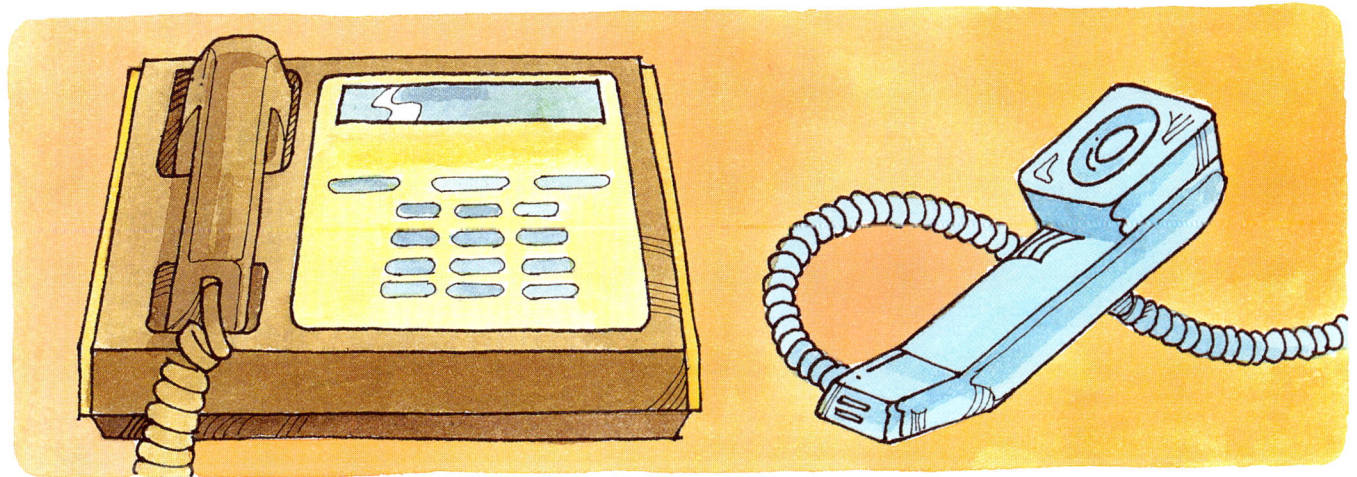

Newspapers
Newspapers are a popular method of communicating daily events. "The Sunday Post" reaches 69 percent of the adults in its home city, the highest readership in the world. In which city is it published?

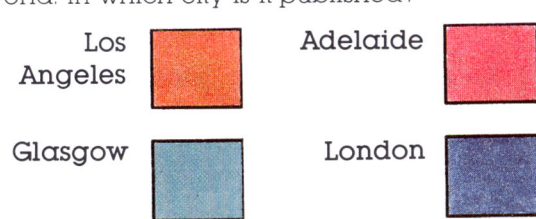

Television
Television allows us to communicate across the world. Our viewing is often interrupted by commercials. By the age of 18, the average American has watched 17,040 hours of television. How many commercials does this include?

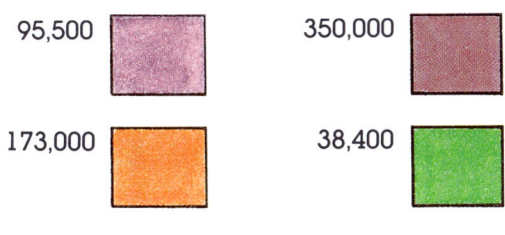

The invention of television made it possible for millions of people to watch a single event at the same time. In 1969, viewers around the world watched man first set foot on the moon. How many people were watching?

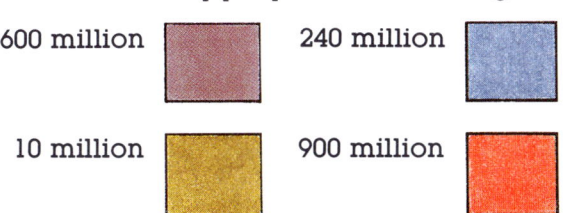

Telephones
The United States has the most telephones in the world. The African country Zaire has the lowest proportion of phones — just one per 1,000 people. How many phones per 1,000 people do Americans have?

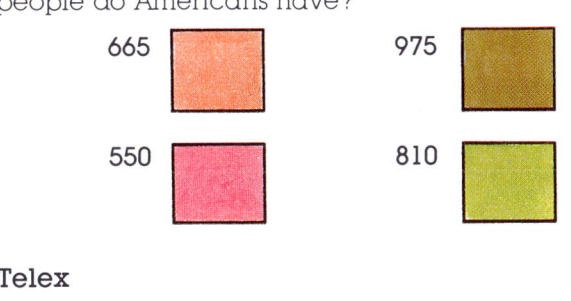

Telex
Sending a telex is like sending a piece of typed information along a telephone line. Messages are sent and received by a special machine. What is it called?

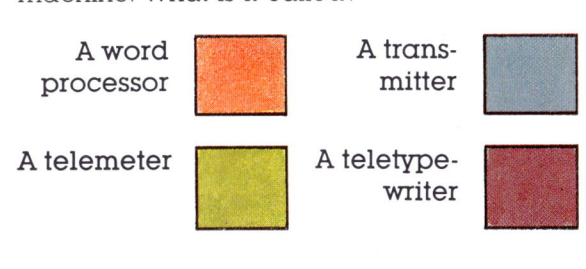

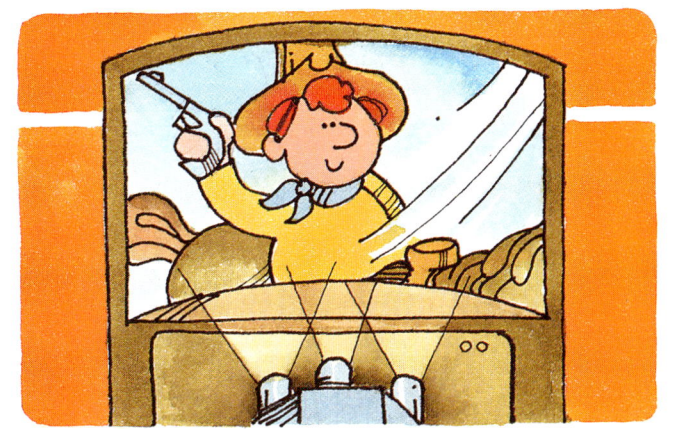

ALTERNATIVE ENERGY

Coal, oil and gas are major sources of energy used to run all kinds of machinery and are vital to our modern way of living. As the world's coal and oil reserves are being used up, we are looking for other sources of energy.

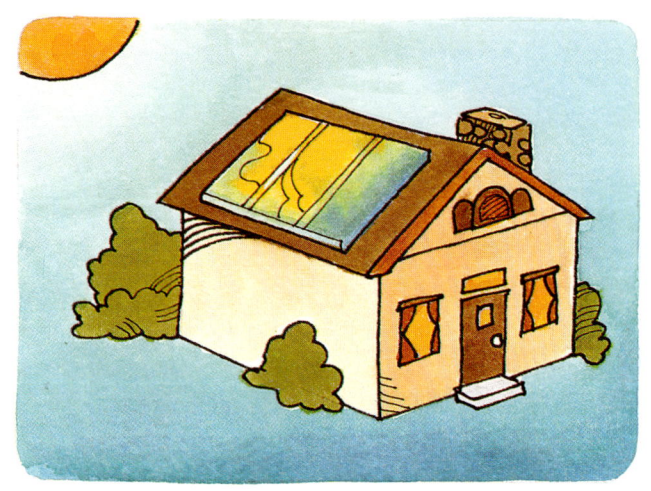

Read each question. Then press **QUESTRON** on the colored square next to the right answer.

Nuclear energy is the result of nuclear fission. Nuclear fission is the name of the process of splitting the nucleus of an atom in two. This releases a burst of energy that is a million times more powerful than the energy released by combustion, the process of burning. What is the nucleus of an atom?

An electron	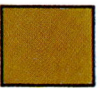	The core	
The shell		The weight	

Hydroelectric power plants supply vast amounts of electricity. They harness a natural element that is freely available in most countries. What is that element?

Fire		Wind	
Lightning		Water	

Electric power was first produced in a nuclear reactor in the U.S.A. In what year?

1951	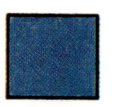	1912	
1960	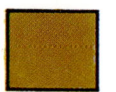	1932	

Light from the sun can be converted into electricity by devices made with two thin layers of silicon. The positive layer contains boron; the negative layer, phosphorus. What are these devices called?

Photo-phobic cells	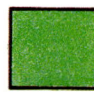	Photo-voltaic cells	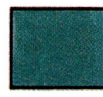
Photo-synthetic cells	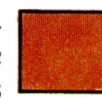	Photo-tropic cells	

Since the seventh century, people have used the force of the wind to generate power in windmills. Today, windmills are often used to pump water from underground wells. Which country is most famous for its windmills?

Denmark		Switzerland	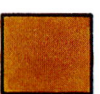
Holland		China	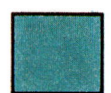

The sun's heat can be collected and used in a variety of ways. Houses can be designed to absorb the sun's heat and store the energy to operate heating and cooling systems. What is this kind of energy called?

Sonar energy		Radiant energy	
Solar energy		Stellar energy	

INTERCEPT!

Heat-seeking missiles from another galaxy have been programmed to hit a power plant. One missile is about to strike! Trace the alien's path with your intercept missile and detonate its charge before it reaches the target.

Track **QUESTRON** through the maze to hit the missile closest to the power plant. But don't stop! There are two more missiles to intercept. Next, strike the second closest missile; finally, strike the third missile to complete your mission.

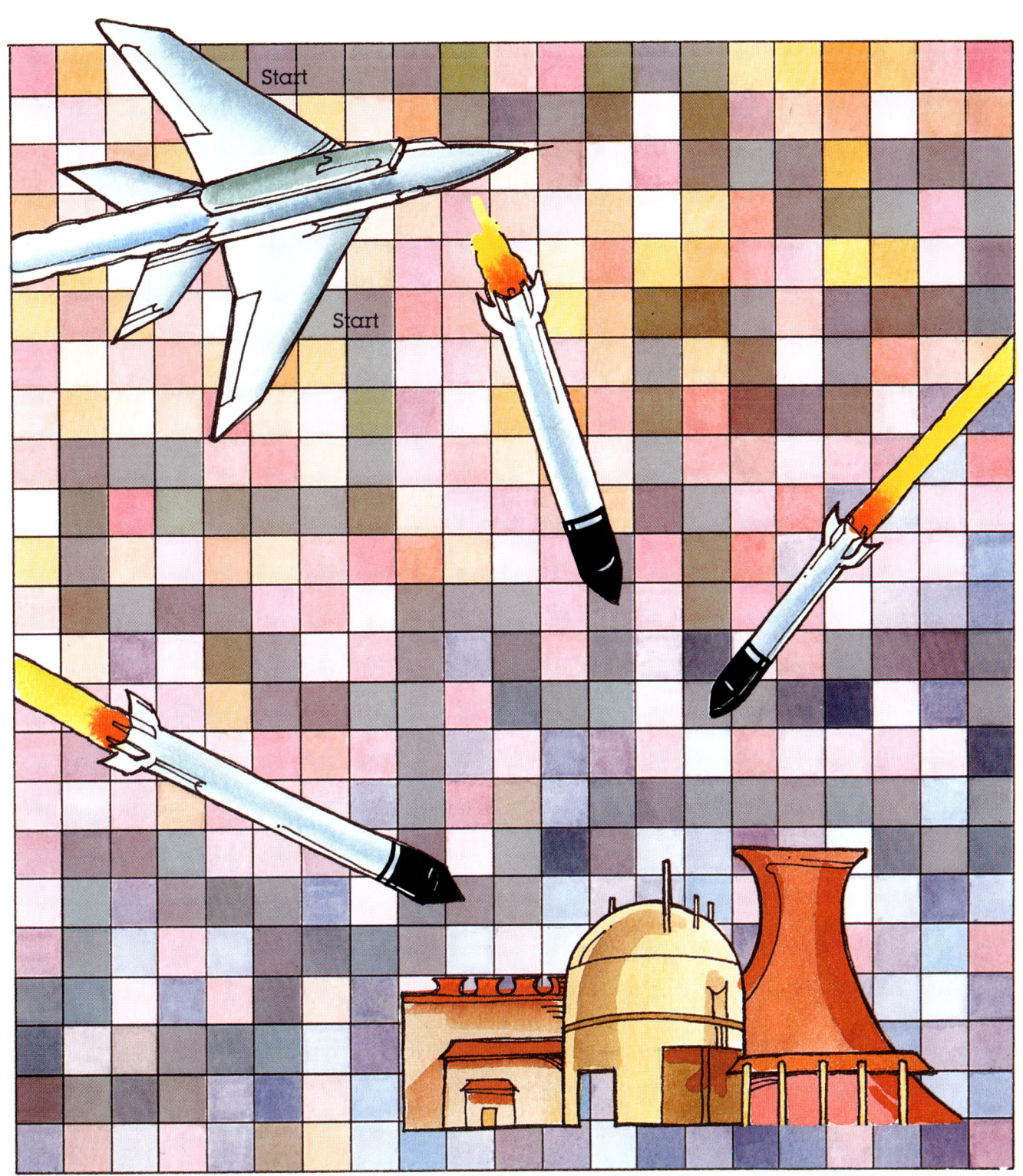

QUICK QUIZ

Track **QUESTRON** through the paths with the correct answers.

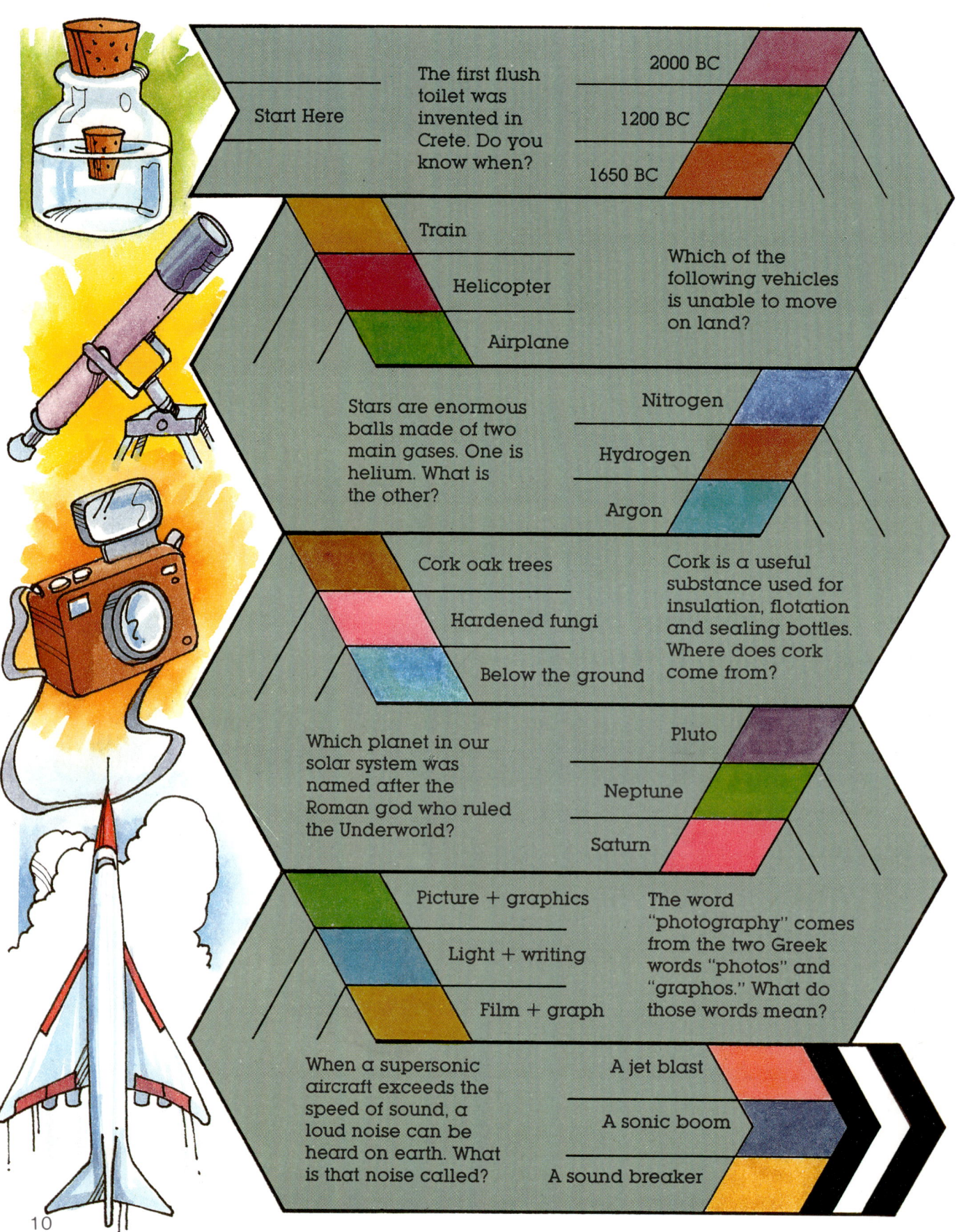

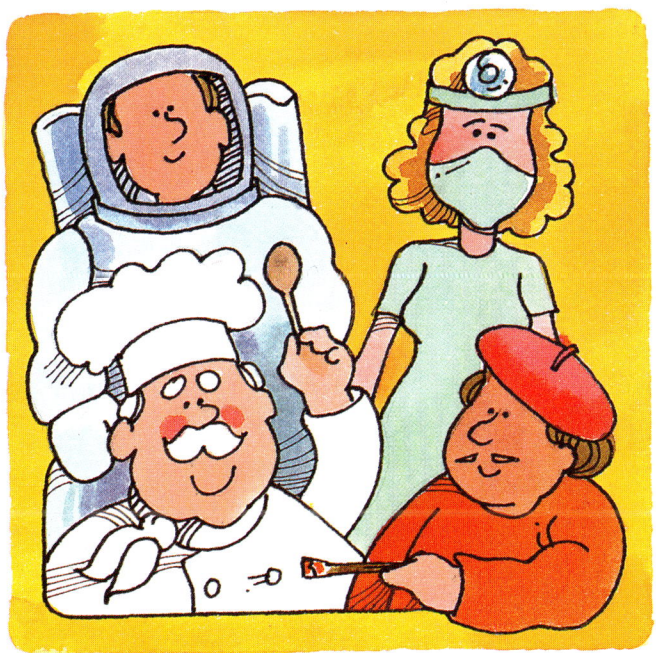

PICK A PROFESSION

You've probably thought about the kind of work you'd eventually like to do. Some people like to work with their hands, others prefer office jobs.

Read each question. Then press **QUESTRON** on the colored square next to the right answer.

Artist

To be successful in any field of art you must first possess natural talent. With proper training that talent can be developed to enable you to work professionally. Some artists work in the fields of advertising, film, television, publishing and music. Others prefer to work independently, selling individual works of art. Which of the following is **not** considered to be an artist?

| Painter | Actor |
| Composer | Agent |

Politician

To be a successful politician you must prove that you really care about your community and your country. You must be good at giving speeches, and you must be loyal and honest. Which well-loved politician smoked large cigars and said these famous words: "We shall never surrender"?

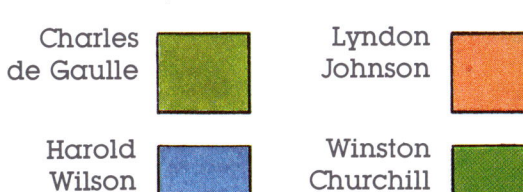

Chef

To become a top chef you must train at a specialized school then work your way through different jobs in a restaurant kitchen to learn every aspect of the profession. Which country is famous for its top class "Cordon Bleu" school of cooking?

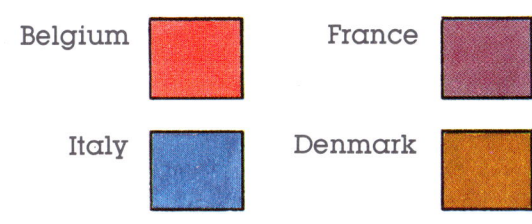

Astronaut

There are fewer than 200 people who can boast this profession! Astronauts are usually chosen from highly skilled pilots and technicians from the armed forces, normally the Air Force. Who was the first astronaut to set foot on the moon?

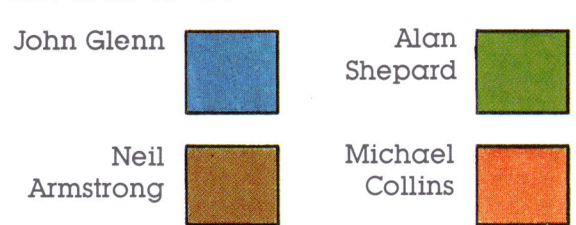

Doctor

There are many areas of medicine in which you can become a specialized doctor. A pediatrician deals with children's problems, an obstetrician specializes in childbirth and a cardiologist is a heart specialist. What does a neurologist specialize in?

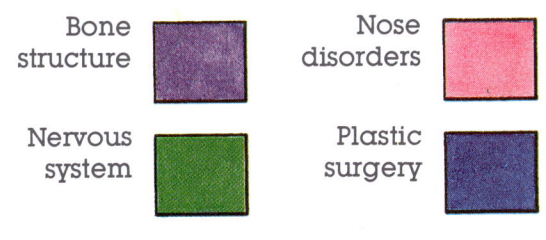

NATURAL RESOURCES

The earth provides us with a wealth of minerals, rocks and fluids that we use for energy, food and prosperity.

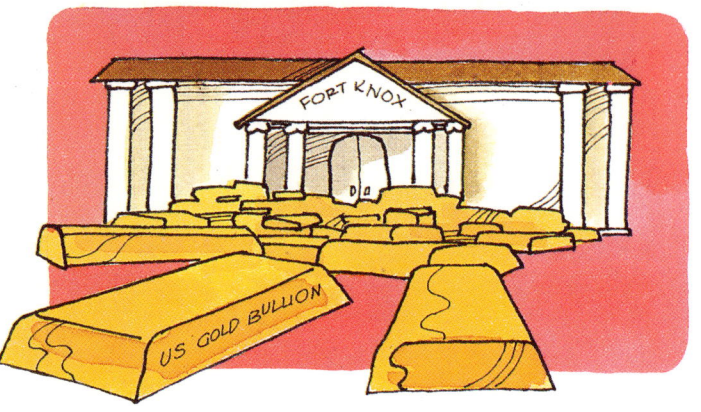

Read each question. Then press **QUESTRON** on the colored square next to the right answer.

Coal
Coal is a marvelous natural fuel. Coal miners have the dangerous task of working hundreds of feet below ground, where they dig out the coal with powerful machines. Coalfields were formed millions of years ago. What is coal made of?

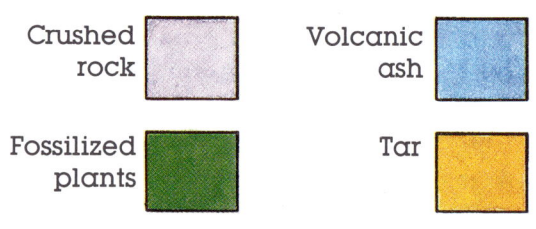

| Crushed rock | Volcanic ash |
| Fossilized plants | Tar |

Iron
Iron is the most used of all metals. During the Iron Age (about 1,000 years BC), people learned how to heat iron to its melting point and mold it into tools and weapons. Thirty-five percent of the world's known iron ore reserves are in one country. Where?

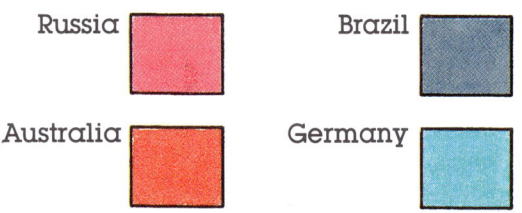

| Russia | Brazil |
| Australia | Germany |

Copper
Copper is a good conductor of heat and is often used to make cooking pots. It can be mixed with another element to make brass. What is the other element used to make brass?

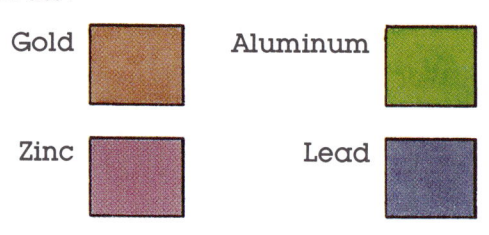

| Gold | Aluminum |
| Zinc | Lead |

Uranium
Uranium is a silvery-white metallic element that is radioactive. It is used in the production of nuclear power. When was uranium first discovered?

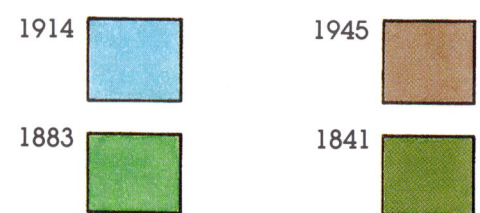

| 1914 | 1945 |
| 1883 | 1841 |

Salt
Salt is naturally present in many of the foods we eat. Many people add extra salt to their food. This is known as common salt. Where do we get common salt from?

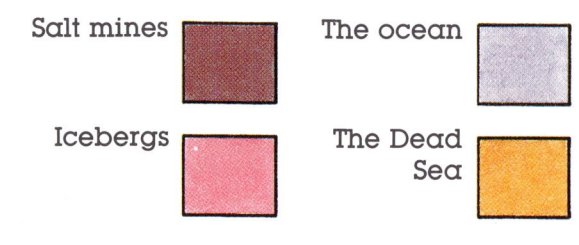

| Salt mines | The ocean |
| Icebergs | The Dead Sea |

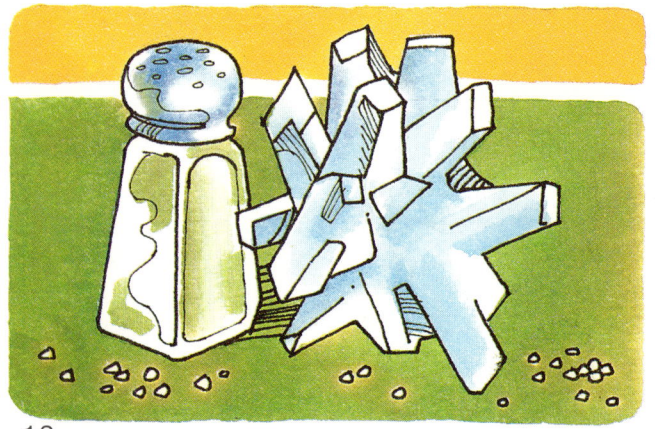

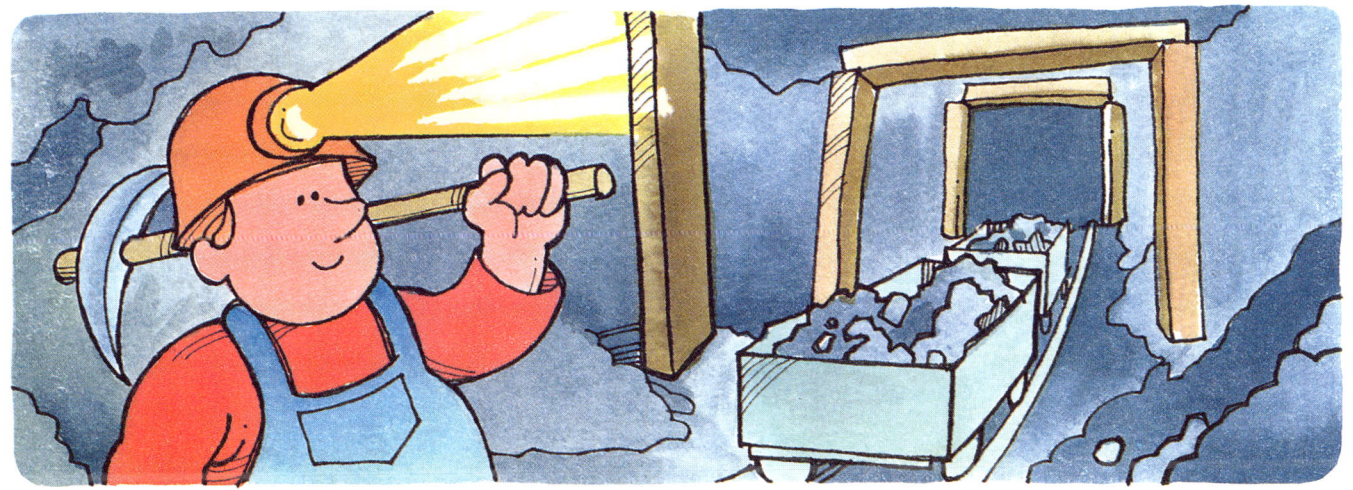

Oil
Oil is perhaps today's most prized natural resource. Countries that possess huge amounts of crude oil have become very wealthy in recent years. Where is the world's largest oil field?

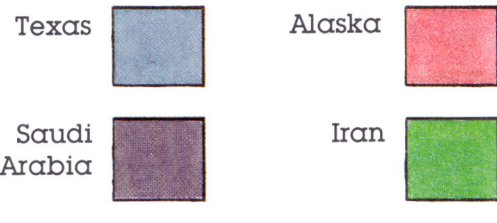

Diamonds
These rare and valuable stones are made of crystallized carbon. The largest diamond in the world was found in 1905 in South Africa. How heavy was it?

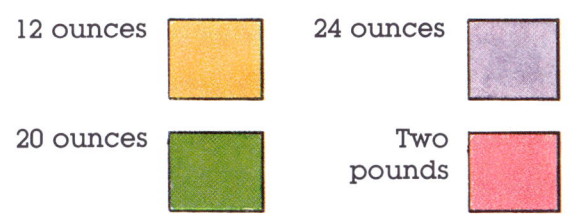

Tin
This very adaptable metal has a low melting point and is used as a protective coating on such items as cans. What is the chemical symbol for tin?

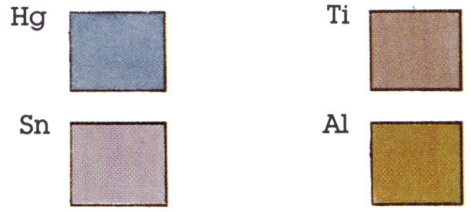

Gold
The largest gold mining area in the world is in South Africa, but the country with the largest gold reserves is the U.S.A. Where is most of the U.S.A.'s gold kept?

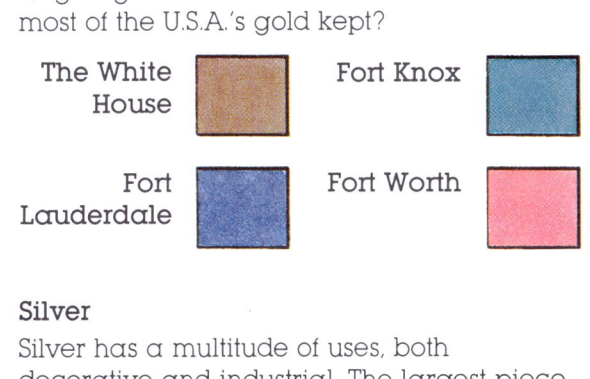

Silver
Silver has a multitude of uses, both decorative and industrial. The largest piece of silver ever mined was found in Mexico over 150 years ago. How heavy was it?

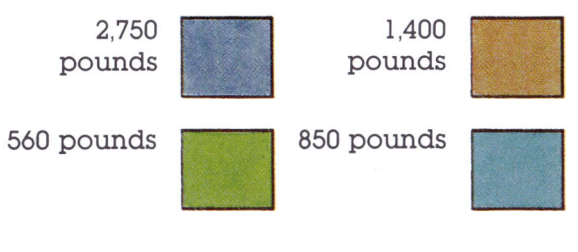

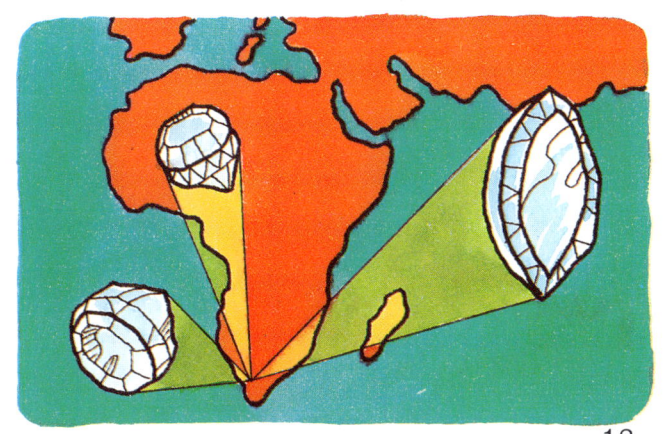

SPACE SHUTTLE

The Space Shuttle is a rocket-powered space craft that, unlike space rockets of the past, can be used over and over. The Space Shuttle program will enable astronauts to build space stations where people can live. A space mission of the future may involve transporting supplies to space stations or taking visitors on tours of outer space.

Here is your mission. Press **QUESTRON** on "Start Here" and blast off from Cape Canaveral, tracking first to Space Station XII to pick up passengers, then to Star Base Delta to drop off supplies. From Delta travel to Saturn to take vapor samples before returning to Edwards Air Force Base in California. Avoid dangerous meteorites.

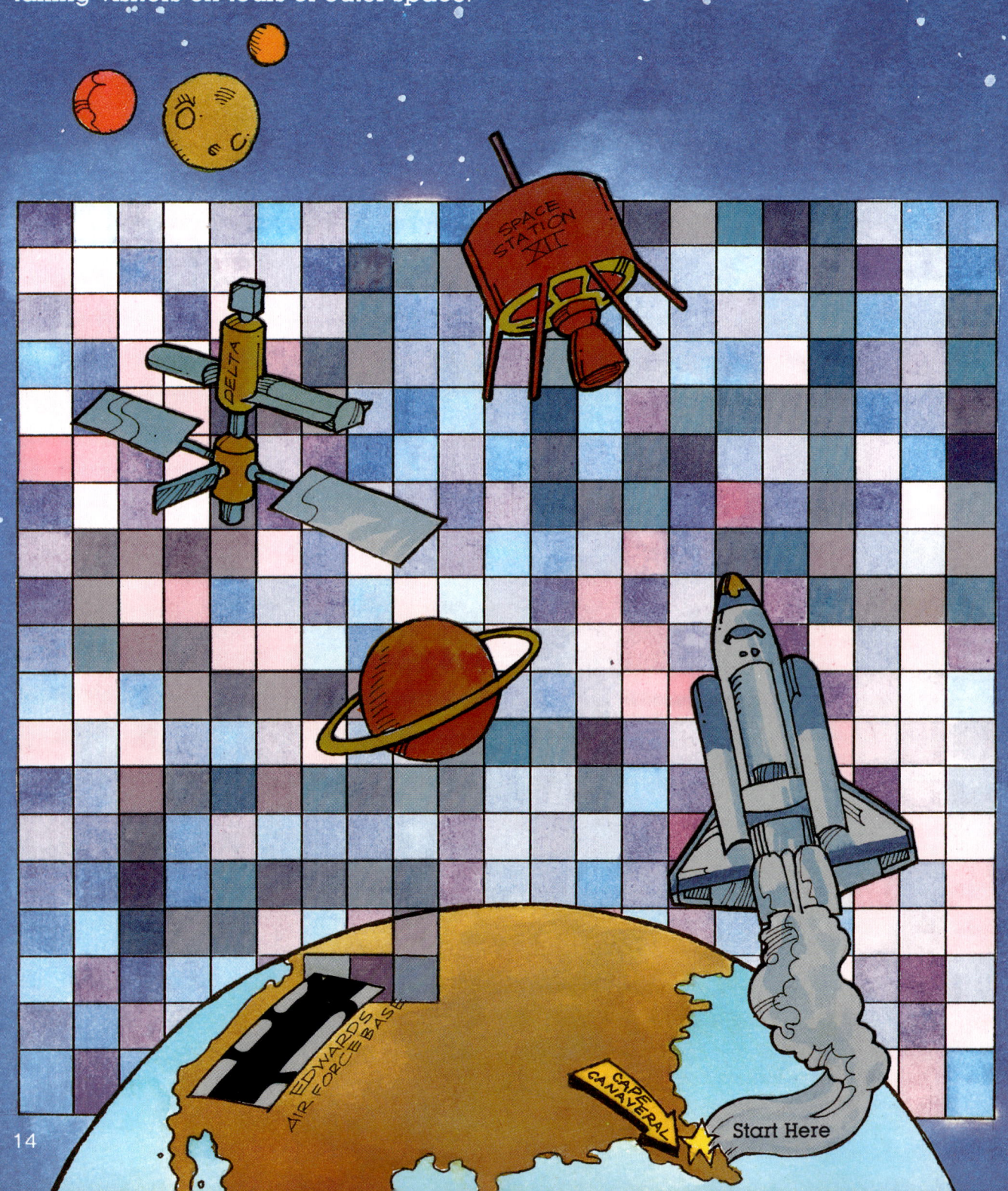

PLANET QUIZ

Of the nine planets in our solar system, Mercury, the fastest moving planet, is closest to the sun. Earth is the third closest planet. Where are the other planets in relation to the sun and to Earth?

Press **QUESTRON** on the colored square next to the right name for each planet.

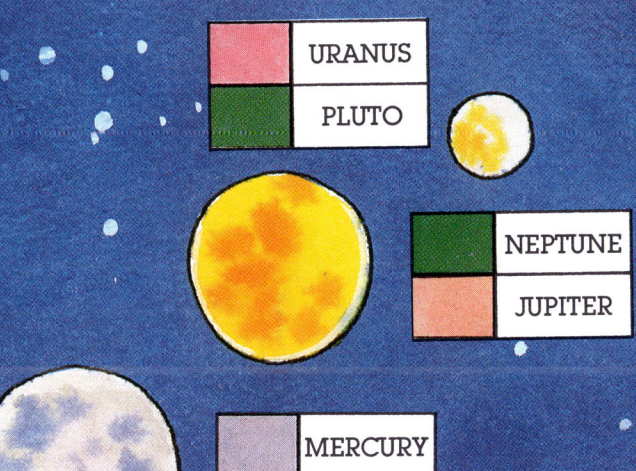
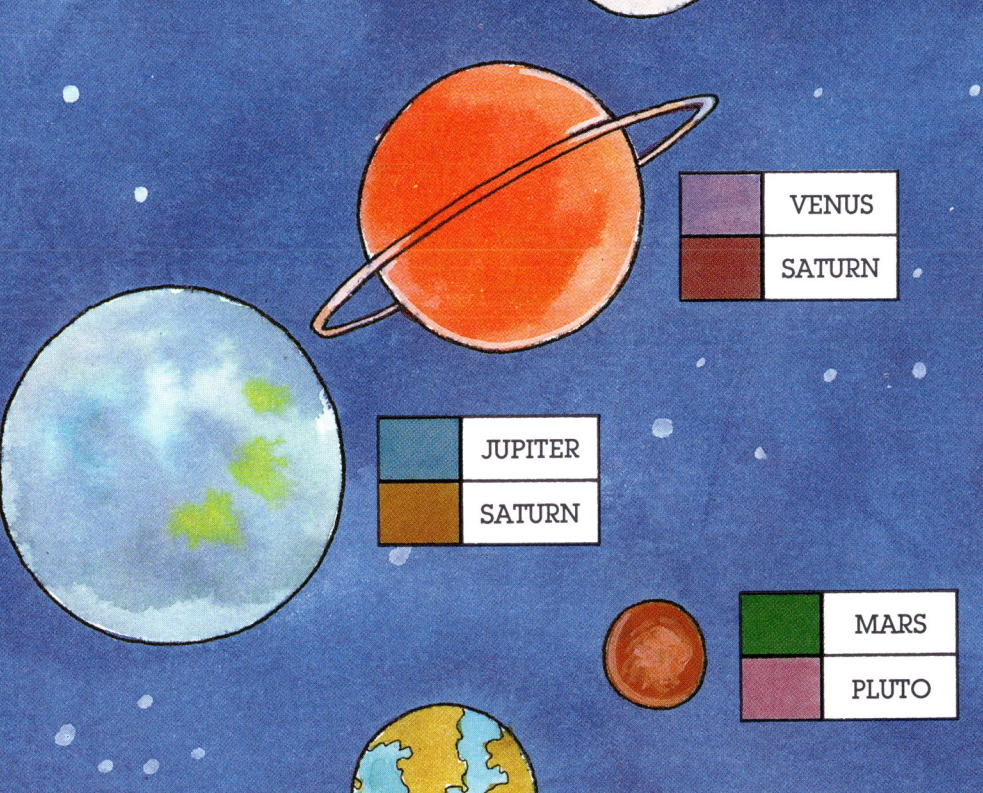
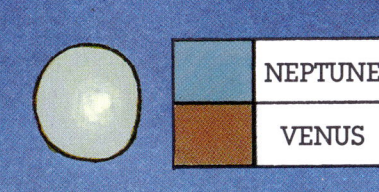

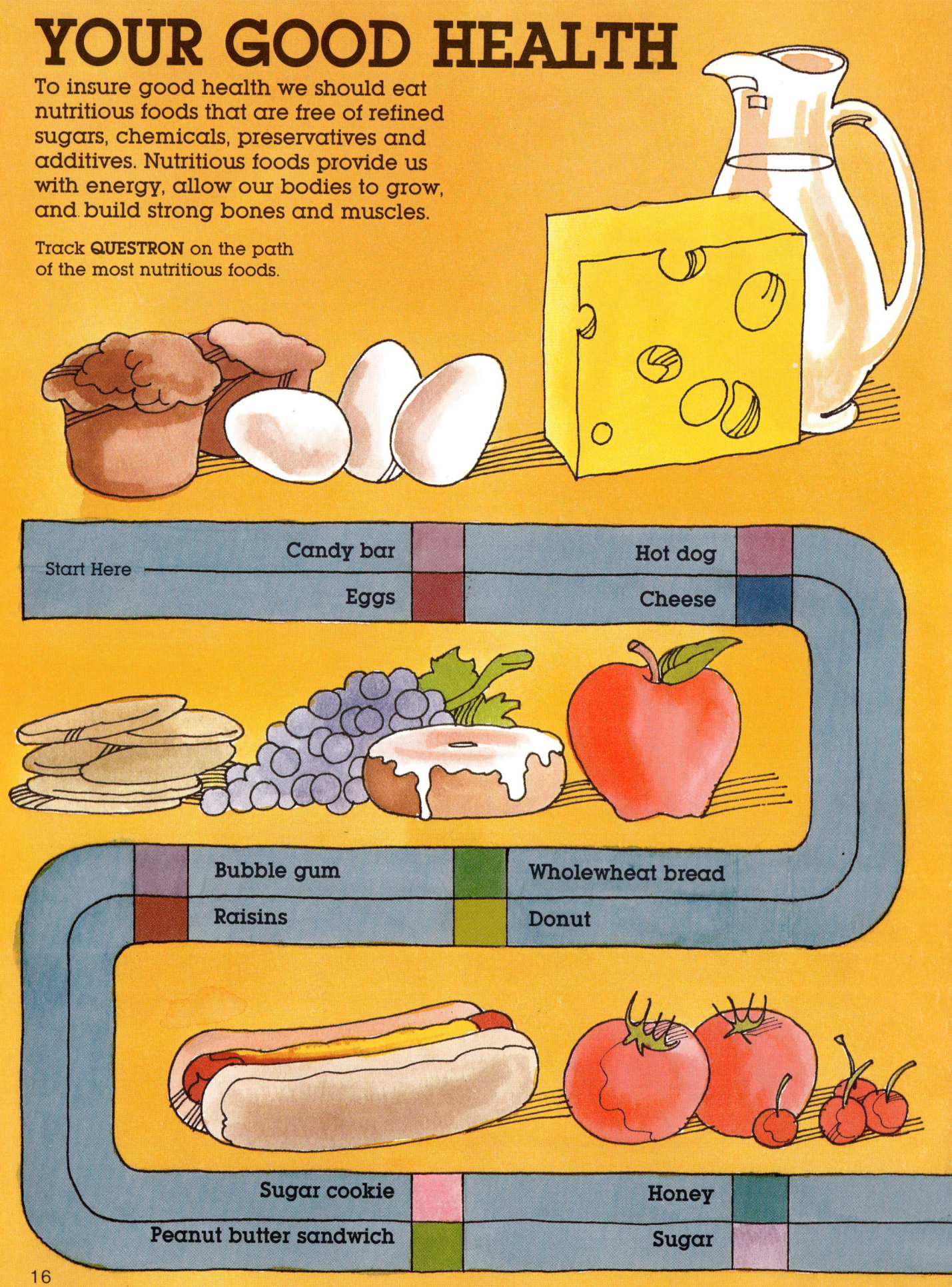

YOUR GOOD HEALTH

To insure good health we should eat nutritious foods that are free of refined sugars, chemicals, preservatives and additives. Nutritious foods provide us with energy, allow our bodies to grow, and build strong bones and muscles.

Track **QUESTRON** on the path of the most nutritious foods.

Start Here — Candy bar — Hot dog
Eggs — Cheese

Bubble gum — Wholewheat bread
Raisins — Donut

Sugar cookie — Honey
Peanut butter sandwich — Sugar

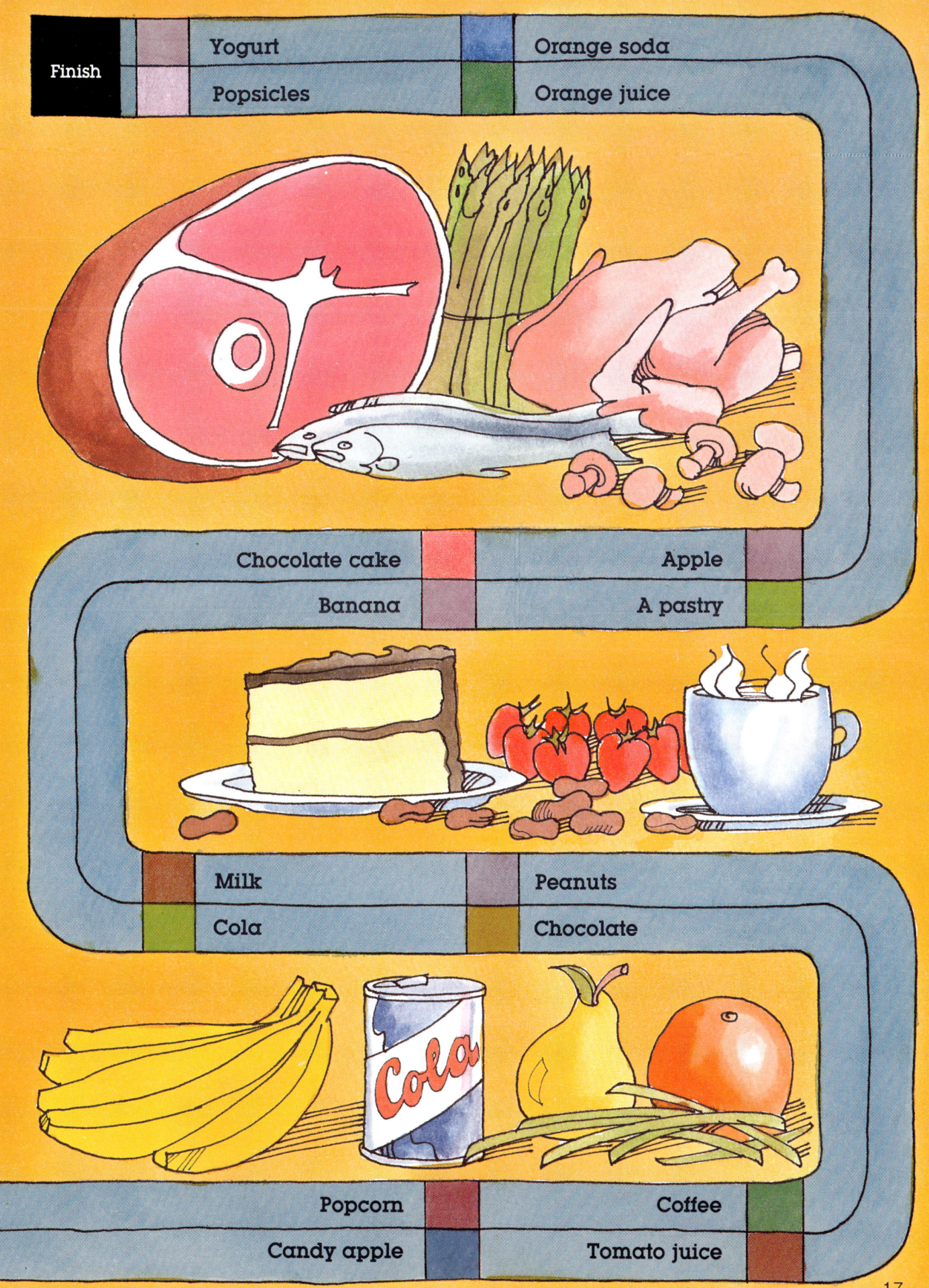

IN THE KITCHEN

Modern kitchens are filled with gadgets and electronic devices that help make household chores easy and enjoyable.

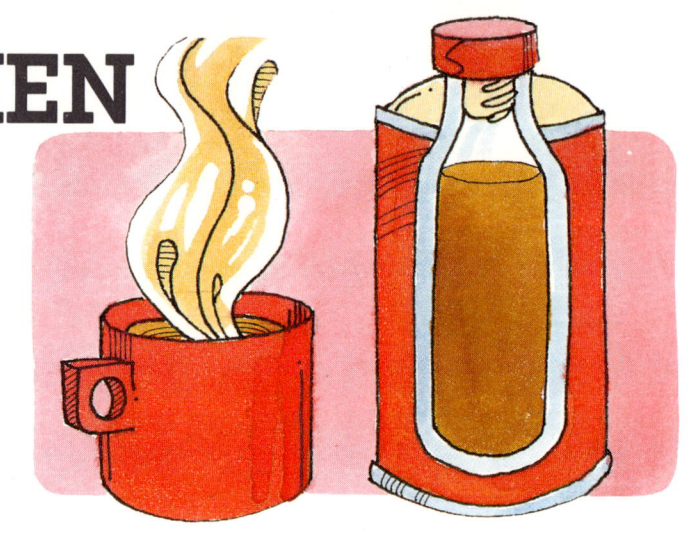

Read each question. Then press QUESTRON on the colored square next to the right answer.

Most foods will last much longer if they are kept in a refrigerator. Foods that are kept in a freezer can be stored for many months, sometimes years. One of the following foods should not be refrigerated if it is to be eaten in its natural state. Which one?

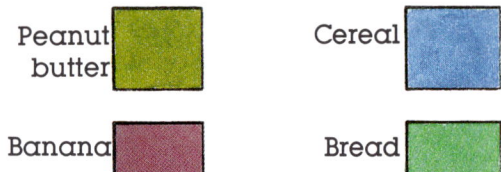

Peanut butter ▢   Cereal ▢
Banana ▢   Bread ▢

Thermostats are often used in kitchen appliances. A thermostat is made by joining two different metals to form a strip. The metals expand at different rates when heated, causing the strip to curve away from an electrical contact. In this way the thermostat switches the electricity off when it reaches a certain temperature. Which of these appliances has a thermostat?

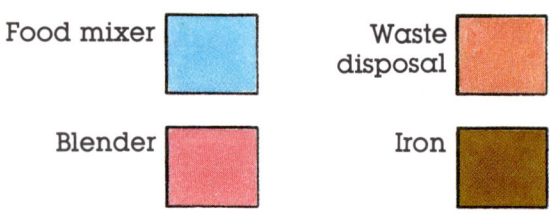

Food mixer ▢   Waste disposal ▢
Blender ▢   Iron ▢

One item we use in the home every day is soap. We use different soaps to clean dishes, clothes, household items and, of course, ourselves. All soaps are made of two basic ingredients. Oil (or fat) is heated and combined with a salty substance obtained from the ashes of plants. What is this substance called?

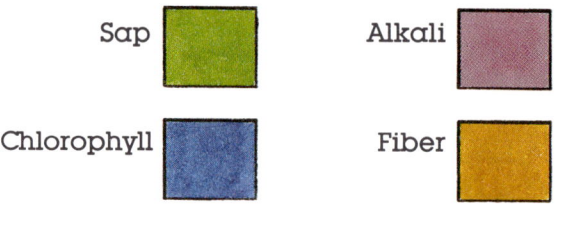

Sap ▢   Alkali ▢
Chlorophyll ▢   Fiber ▢

What is the special name given to the kitchen in a boat or a plane?

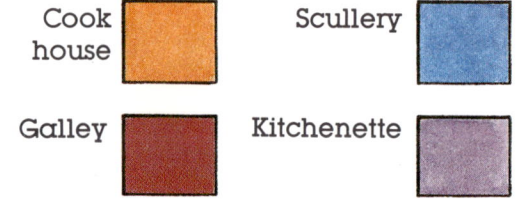

Cook house ▢   Scullery ▢
Galley ▢   Kitchenette ▢

Dishwashers have taken over the job of washing all those dishes we use. Cups, saucers, mugs and plates are usually made of earthenware. Earthenware dishes can be used over and over, and will withstand extremes of temperature. What is earthenware made from?

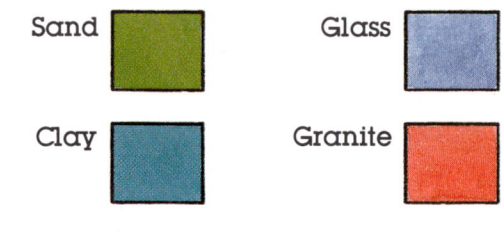

Sand ▢   Glass ▢
Clay ▢   Granite ▢

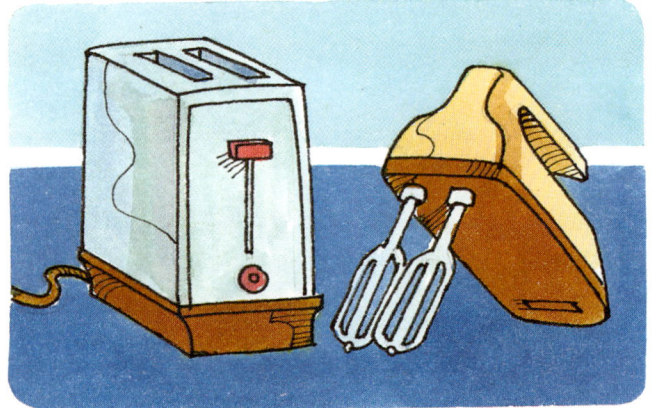

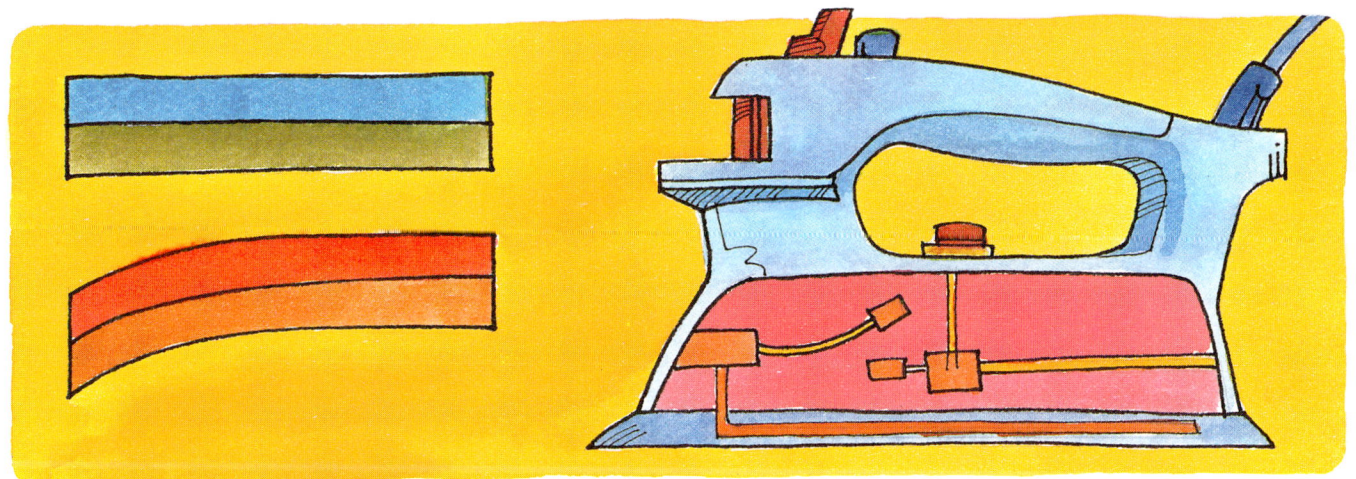

Vinegar is a sour liquid that can be made from wine. It is used in a variety of dressings and is a useful preservative. The word "vinegar" comes from the French "vin" meaning "wine", and "aigre" meaning "sour". The main ingredient in vinegar is a specific kind of acid. What is it called?

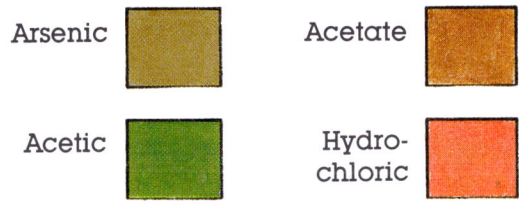

One of the first things we learn to make in the kitchen is pastry. Pastry is a simple dough that is used as a crust for pies and tarts. There are three main ingredients in pastry: flour, shortening (fat), and . . .

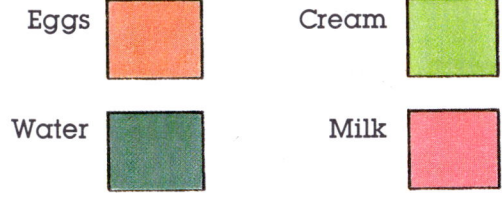

Microwave ovens enable us to cook food faster than any other method. High-frequency waves pass through food and agitate the food molecules, causing high frictional heat. This internal heat cooks the food in minutes. What are microwaves?

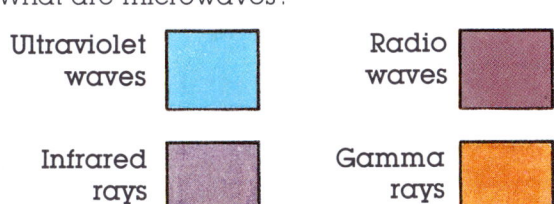

Vaccum flasks keep food and drinks hot (or cold) for hours without the help of a heat source. Heat conduction is prevented by a double-layered glass container. The vacuum between the layers prevents heat escaping by convection, and a silvering on the glass prevents heat escaping by another method. What method is that?

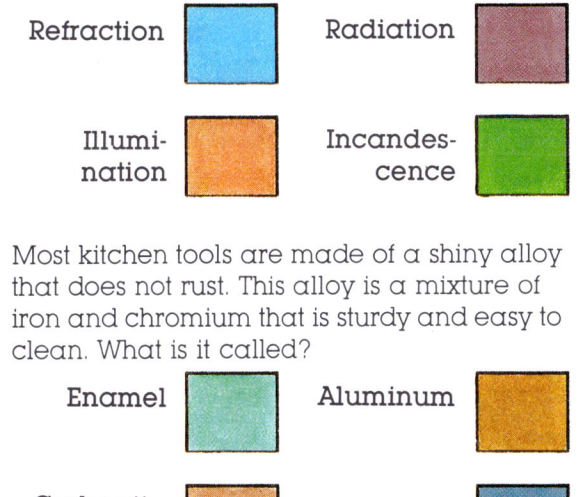

Most kitchen tools are made of a shiny alloy that does not rust. This alloy is a mixture of iron and chromium that is sturdy and easy to clean. What is it called?

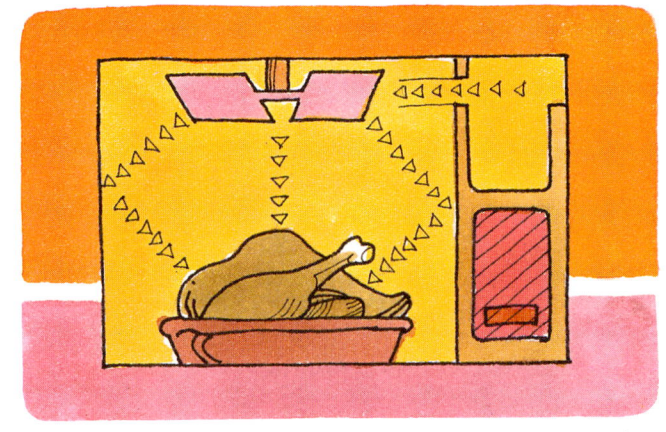

BUILD-A-BIKE

Although designs for a bicycle were first drawn by Leonardo da Vinci, in 1493, the first bicycle was not built until 1840.

See if you can build a modern bicycle. Track **QUESTRON** through the maze and collect the bicycle parts in the following order: FRAME, HANDLEBARS, SADDLE, WHEELS, PEDALS, CHAIN.

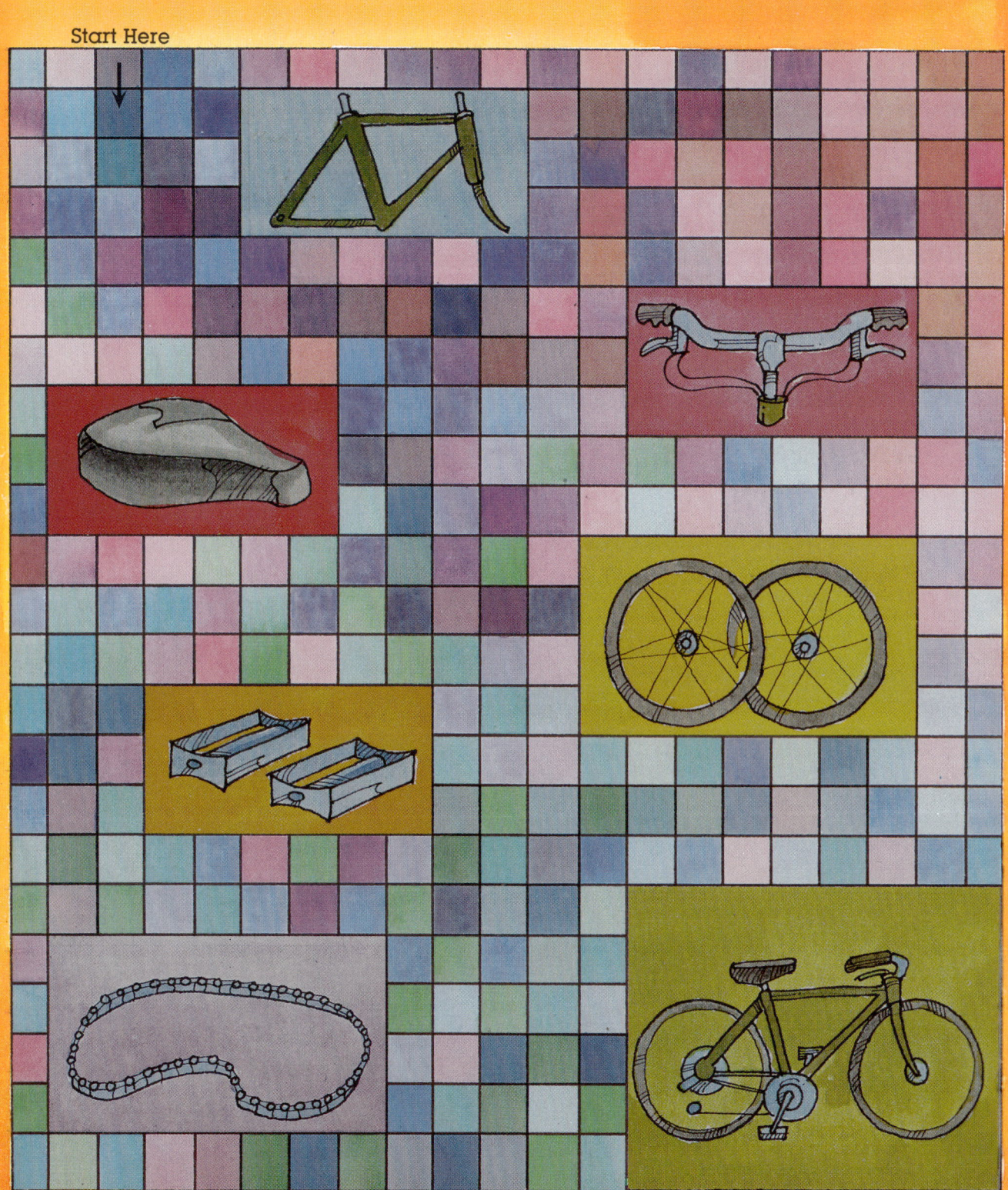

TRIATHLON

A triathlon is a strenuous contest requiring great physical strength and endurance. Contestants must swim 2.4 miles, bicycle 112 miles and run 26.2 miles without stopping. The world record, set in 1983, is nine hours, 20 minutes.

Track **QUESTRON** through the triathlon course to the finish line.

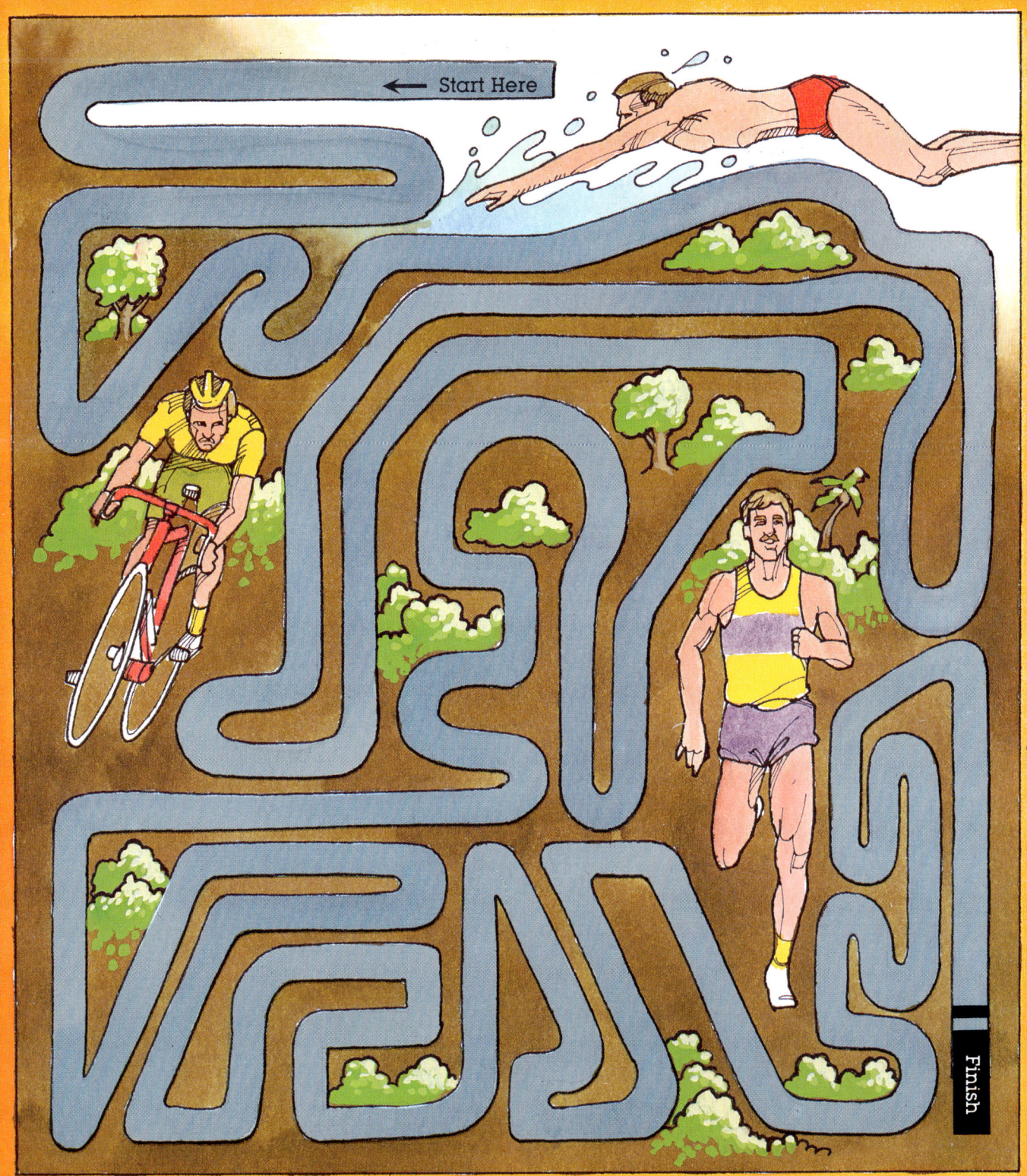

WEATHER

Our year is divided into four seasons: spring, summer, autumn and winter. Each season suggests a particular kind of weather. For most of the world's population winters are cold and cloudy, summers are warm and sunny; but the people who live near the equator have hot weather all year.

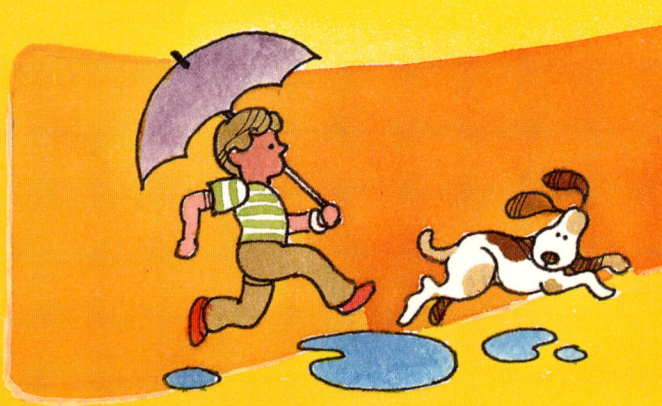

Read each question. Then press **QUESTRON** on the colored square next to the right answer.

In the days of sailing ships, sailors who traveled the great oceans of the world depended on the strong winds that blow toward the equator. These winds blow from about the 30th parallels north and south of the equator. What are they called?

Westerly winds   The mistral

The doldrums 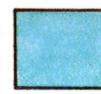   Trade winds

Tidal waves are not related to real tides. They are caused by undersea earthquakes or by distant hurricanes. Tidal waves are also known by a Japanese name — "tsunami". What does it mean?

Giant breaker 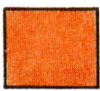   Swift tide

High roller    Storm wave

Tornadoes are swirling tunnels of air that can suck large obstacles off the ground. They are caused when an updraft of air hits a wind current blowing in the opposite direction. How fast can the swirling air travel?

450 m.p.h. 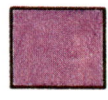   300 m.p.h.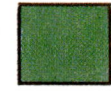

700 m.p.h. 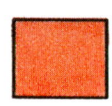   600 m.p.h.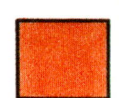

Clouds in the sky can mean there is a chance of rain, but not all clouds are made of moist air alone. Heavily populated or industrial cities often have a cloud layer that is produced by smoke and pollution. What is this polluted cloud layer called?

Smog 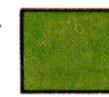   Haze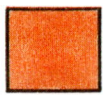

Drizzle    Smut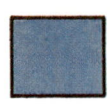

When there is a sudden drop in temperature, the water particles in the air condense and cling to specks of dust. Together, these specks produce the haze we call fog. Which of these cities is famous for fog?

Paris    Sydney

San Francisco 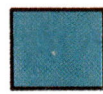   Dallas

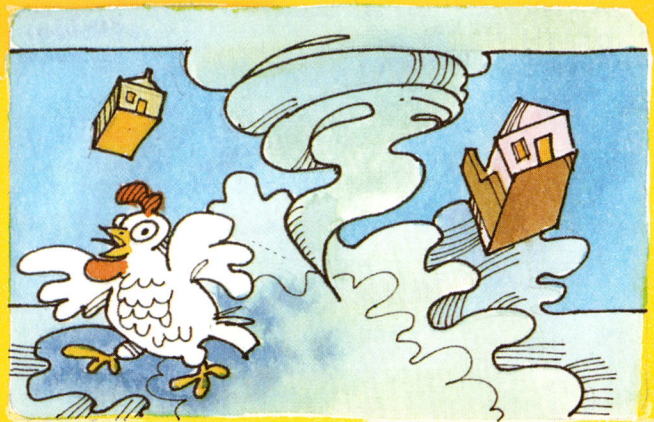

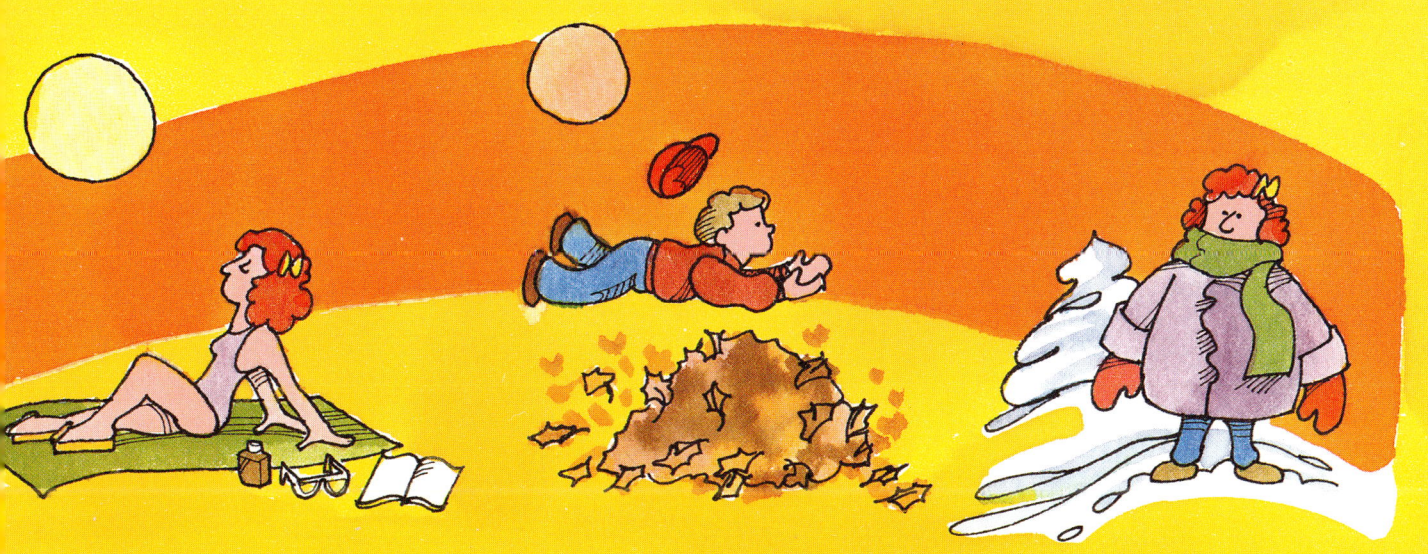

The Gulf Stream is a warm ocean current that starts in the Caribbean Sea and travels thousands of miles across the Atlantic Ocean. The warm winds that blow off the Gulf Stream help raise winter temperatures in certain countries. Which of the following countries benefits from the warming effects of the Gulf Stream?

United Kingdom    Greece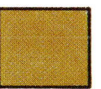

Finland    Italy

Every place on earth has its own climate. An area's climate is the average type of weather that a particular location gets. When describing climate, scientists consider two factors. One is precipitation (rain, snow, etc.). What is the other factor?

Pressure    Daylight

Temperature    Population

In North America, the greatest amount of snow to accumulate in one season was 25 feet 5 inches deep. Where did it fall?

Nebraska 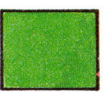   Ontario

Alaska 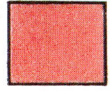   Washington State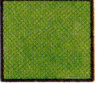

Earthquakes occur when two land masses that normally slide past each other very slowly become locked. If the force is too great, the rocks break and shift, causing a sudden jolt. The force of an earthquake is measured on a scale of numbers. What is that scale called?

Barometer 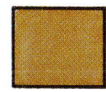   Sliding

Richter    Metric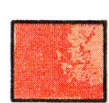

Hurricanes, also known as cyclones and typhoons, are storms that create winds over 75 m.p.h. In 1980 a hurricane tore through the Caribbean at 185 m.p.h. What was its name?

Allen    Camille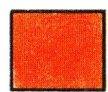

Betsy    David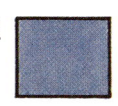

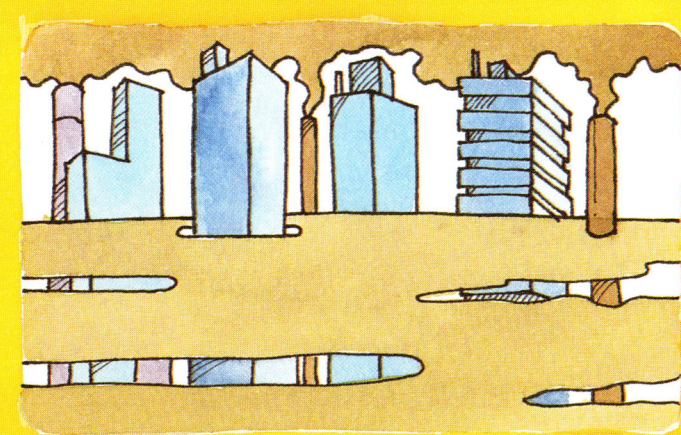

EUREKA!

All the day-to-day objects that we take for granted took scientists and scholars years to discover or develop. Major inventions of this century include television, telephones, motion pictures, transistors and jet propulsion.

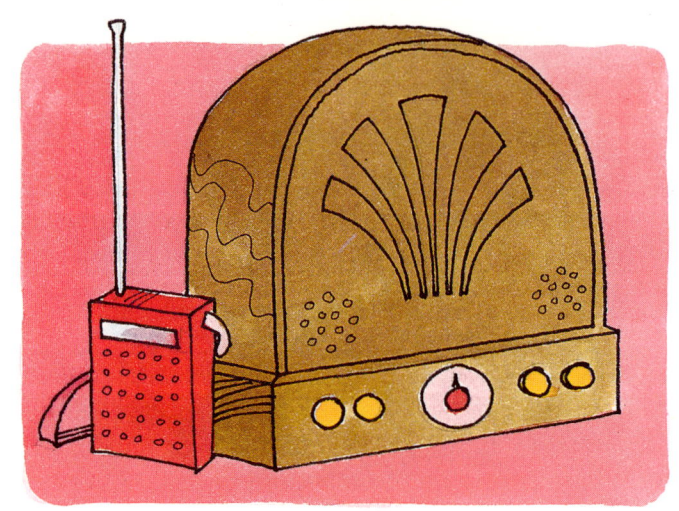

Read each question. Then press **QUESTRON** on the colored square next to the right answer.

Radio
Radios can receive signals transmitted by electrical waves without the use of wires. Early radios were known as wirelesses. The first wireless was invented by Guglielmo Marconi in 1895. What was his nationality?

| Spanish ■ | Hungarian ■ |
| Italian ■ | Welsh ■ |

Penicillin
Antibiotics are used to combat a variety of diseases. Although Louis Pasteur first discovered their benefits in 1887, today's best-known antibiotic, penicillin, was not produced until 1928. Who discovered penicillin?

| Jonas Salk ■ | Alexander Fleming ■ |
| Carl Anderson ■ | Leon Foucault ■ |

Safety Match
Compared to the discovery of fire, the match is a very new invention. The first safety match was developed in 1845 by J. E. Lundstrom. Which country was he from?

| Norway ■ | Finland ■ |
| Denmark ■ | Sweden ■ |

Ferris Wheel
The first Ferris wheel measured 250 feet in diameter and had 36 cars, each with 60 seats. It could hold 2,160 people! Named after its inventor, George Ferris, it was completed in 1893. Where was it located?

| Coney Island ■ | Paris ■ |
| Berlin ■ | Chicago ■ |

Light Bulb
Every light bulb has three basic parts — a filament, a bulb and a base. Electricity is fed to the filament, which gives off light when heated. The electric light bulb was invented in 1879. Who was the inventor?

| Alexander Graham Bell ■ | Thomas Edison ■ |
| Galileo ■ | Marie Curie ■ |

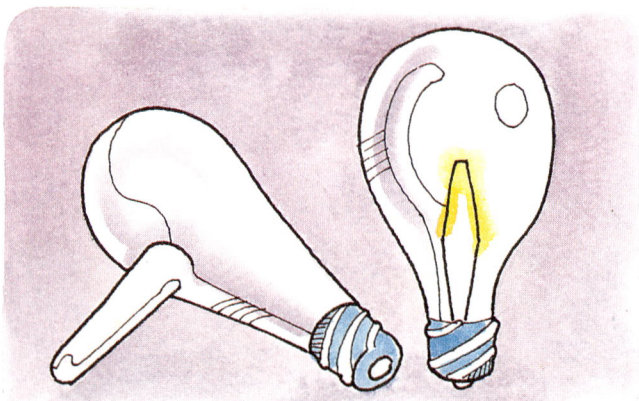

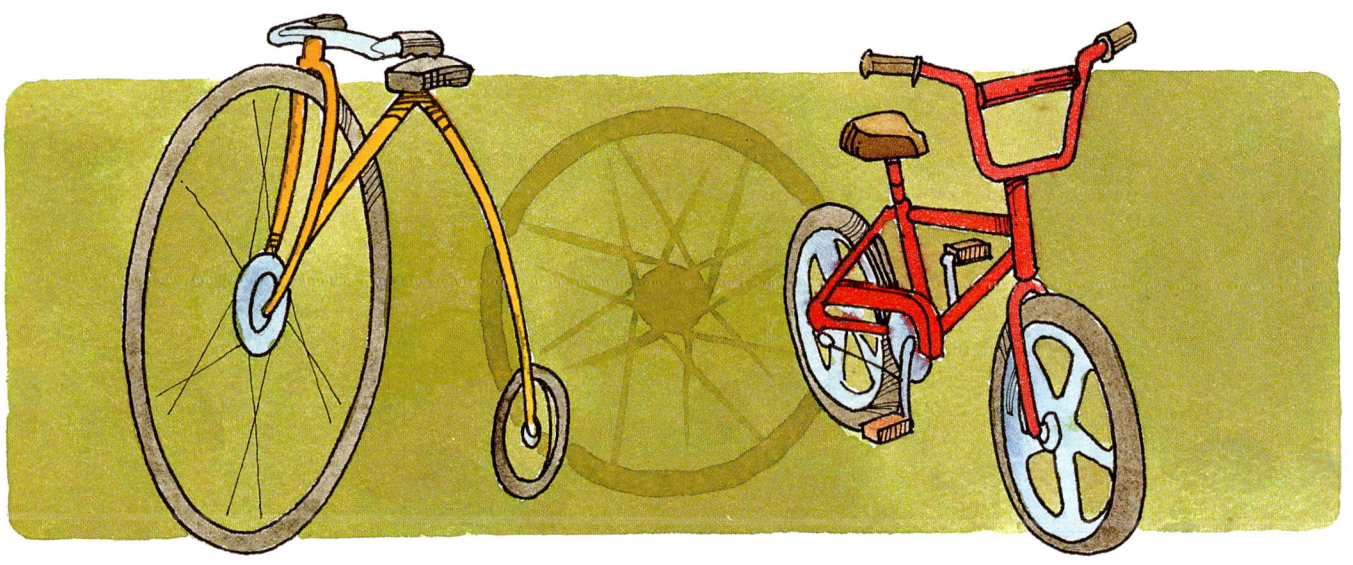

Nylon
Many of our clothes are made from nylon, which was first developed by Wallace Carothers in 1935. What is nylon made from?

Shredded vines 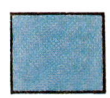		Mixed chemicals 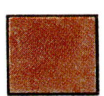	
Animal fur 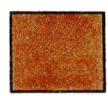		Compressed paper	

Automobile
The first gasoline-driven car was built by Karl Friedrich Benz in 1885. Although this is the first accepted car, a small car was built in 1668 by Ferdinand Verbiest, a Jesuit priest. How was his car powered?

By gas 		By steam 	
By oil 		By electricity	

Watch
A German locksmith, Peter Henlein, is credited with making the first watch. In the early 1500s he invented a mainspring to power clocks. Around 1504 he made a small portable clock in the form of a pocket watch. How were clocks driven before Henlein invented the mainspring?

By electricity 		By batteries 	
By falling weights 		By solar energy 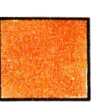	

Bicycle
The first designs for a bicycle were drawn by Leonardo da Vinci in 1493. A French nobleman, Comte Mede de Sivrac, built a crude bike in 1790. The first accepted bicycle was built by a Scotsman, Kirkpatrick Macmillan. When was it completed?

1840 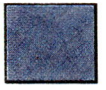		1800 	
1911 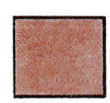		1760 	

Laser Beam
Lasers emit a penetrating light beam and are used in a variety of ways, including delicate surgery. T.H. Maiman of the U.S. created the first working laser. When?

1960 		1933 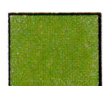	
1971 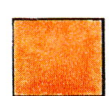		1922 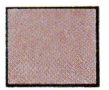	

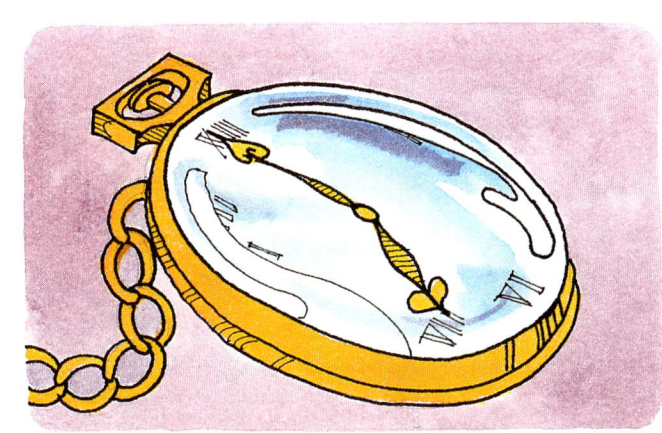

BULLET TRAIN

Today's high speed passenger trains have become very popular with people who work in big cities, but prefer to live in country areas. These trains enable people to travel quickly and avoid the traffic problems so often caused by cars.

See how fast you can answer the questions as you travel on the bullet train. Track the correct answers with **QUESTRON**.

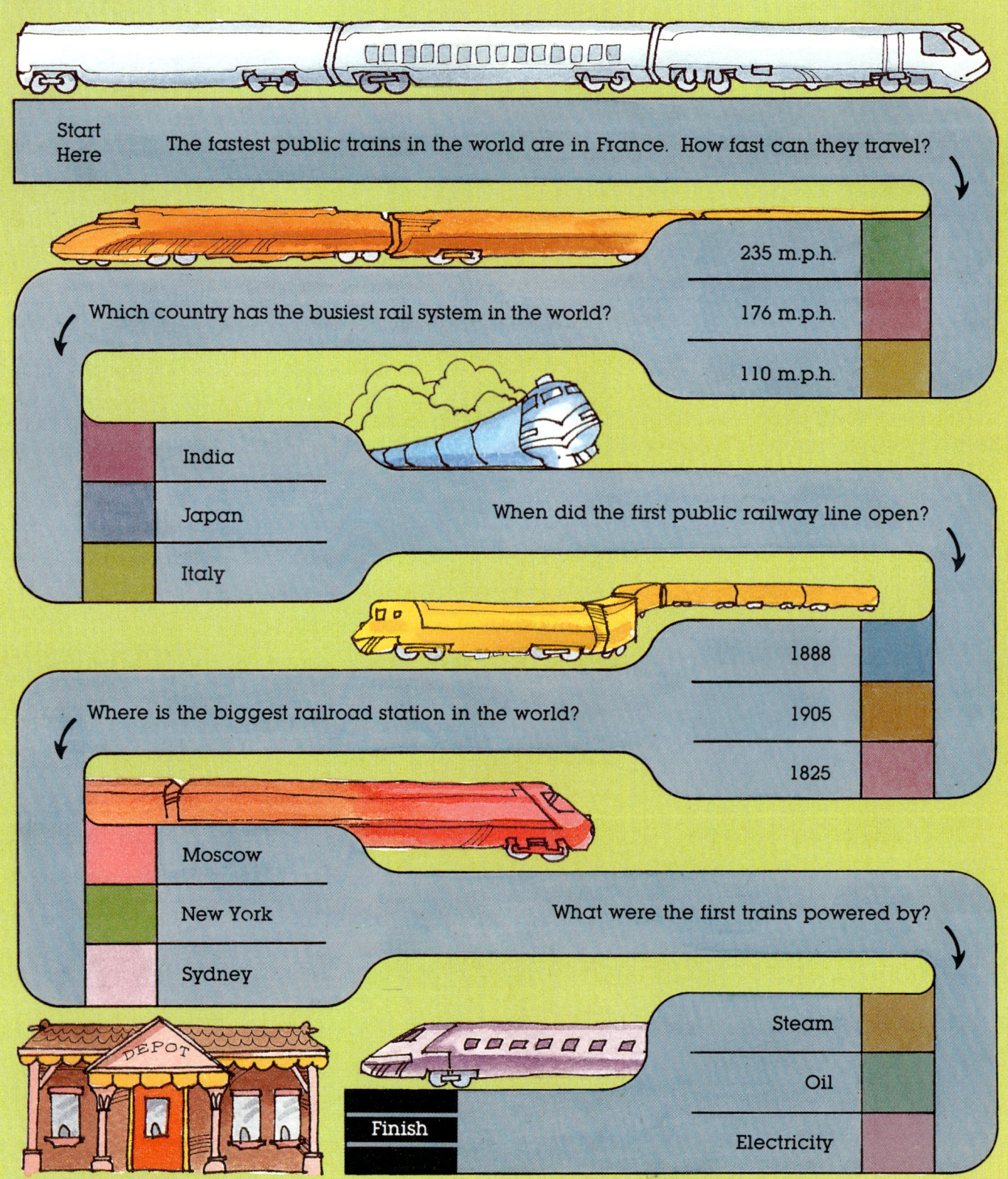

Start Here — The fastest public trains in the world are in France. How fast can they travel?

- 235 m.p.h.
- 176 m.p.h.
- 110 m.p.h.

Which country has the busiest rail system in the world?

- India
- Japan
- Italy

When did the first public railway line open?

- 1888
- 1905
- 1825

Where is the biggest railroad station in the world?

- Moscow
- New York
- Sydney

What were the first trains powered by?

- Steam
- Oil
- Electricity

Finish

26

FREIGHT TRAIN

The longest freight train on record was 3.5 miles long and consisted of 450 cars. It was pulled by three diesels in the front and pushed by five diesels from behind. The train was filled with coal and weighed 44,555 tons.

Track **QUESTRON** from the coalfield to the freight yard. Do not cross any red signals.

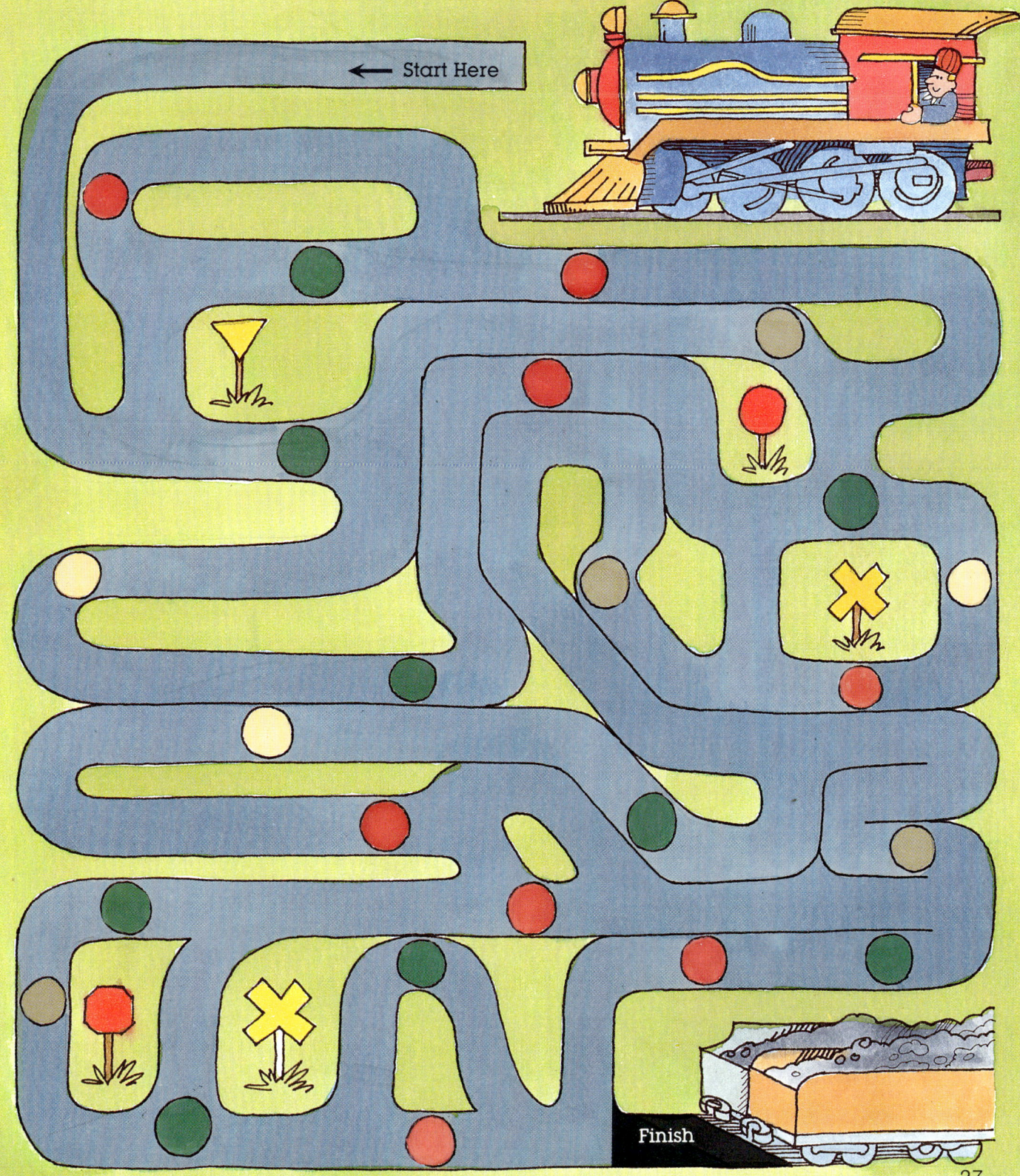

OUTER SPACE

To our early ancestors, space was a void dotted with distant lights. The mysteries of the heavens were then explained through myths and folk tales. With the invention of the telescope, we began to understand the stars and planets. With the development of space travel, we have taken our first steps toward them.

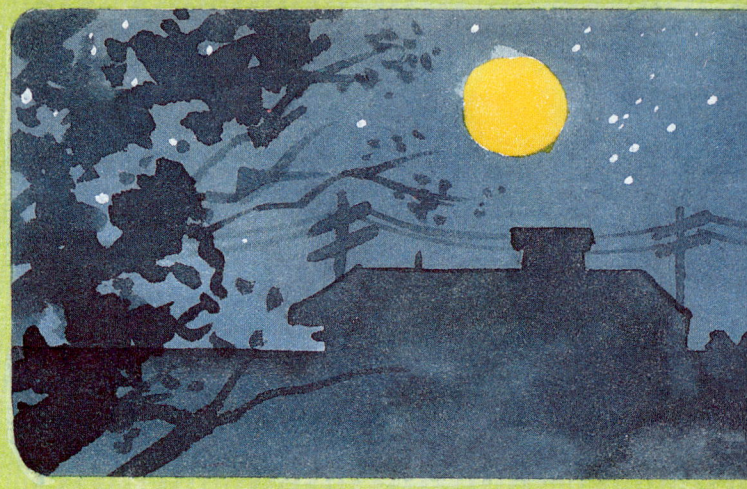

Read each question. Then press **QUESTRON** on the colored square next to the right answer.

Earth's atmosphere is divided into five layers. The outer four layers are often referred to by one name. What is it?

Ozono-sphere		Ionosphere	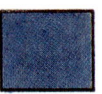
Remo-sphere	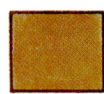	Horisphere	

Scientists discovered a chemical element in space long before we knew it existed on Earth. Which element is it?

Nitrogen	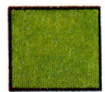	Helium	
Aluminum	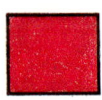	Sulfur	

Earth belongs to a family of nine major planets known as the solar system. Every planet in our solar system revolves around the sun in the same direction. Which planet is farthest from the sun?

Pluto		Uranus	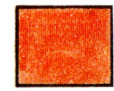
Jupiter	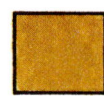	Mars	

The sun is a star that produces energy which makes it shine. It is also extremely hot. The heat it generates keeps everything on Earth alive. Compared to other stars, the sun is only average in size. What is the sun's diameter?

864,000 miles		85,100 miles	
275,000 miles	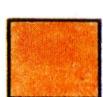	682,000 miles	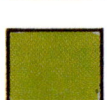

Jupiter is so large it can hold 1,000 Earths. It rotates rapidly and has 13 moons. Jupiter is known for its Great Red Spot, which is 13,000 miles wide. What is this spot?

Burning gases	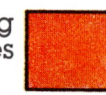	A fiery moon	
A meteor shower		A storm	

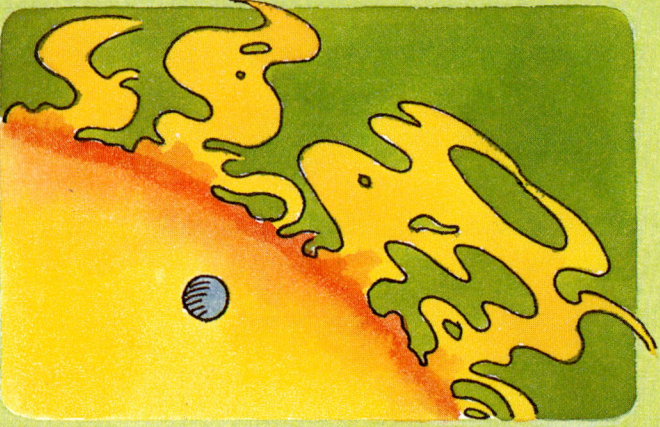

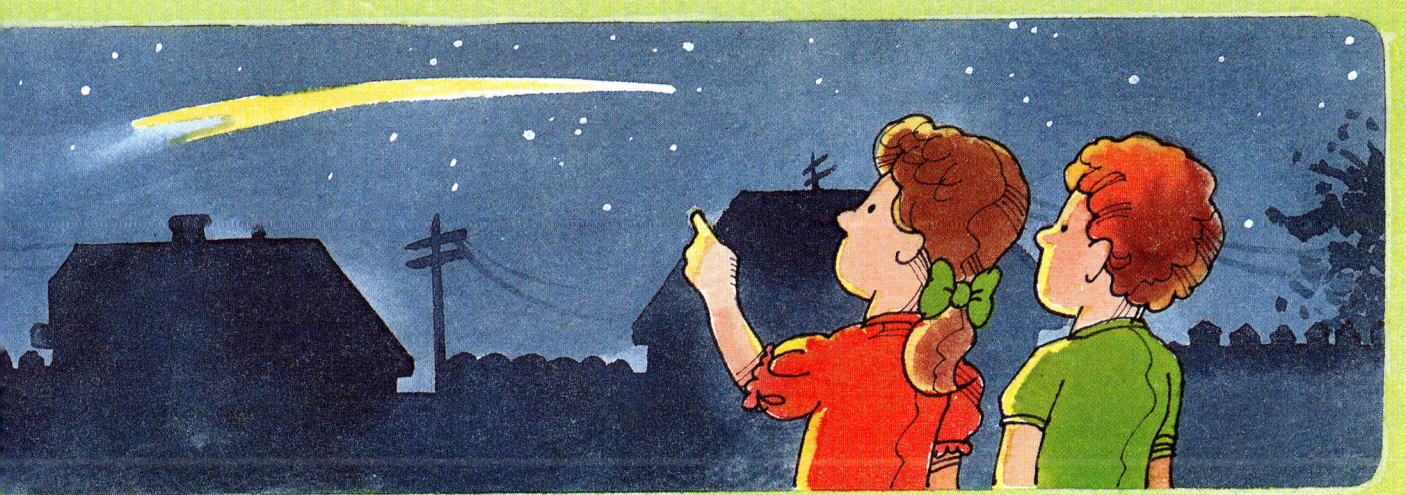

We know more about the planet Mars than any other planet except our own. In 1971 an American spacecraft was able to photograph all of Mars. What was the spacecraft called?

Mariner 9    Voyager 1

Pioneer 10   Viking 2

The planet Mercury was named after the Roman messenger god. It is the fastest moving planet in orbit and takes 88 days to revolve around the sun. (Earth takes 365 days.) How fast does Mercury travel?

1,451 m.p.h. 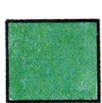   1,068 m.p.h.

88 m.p.h.    107,000 m.p.h.

An infrared astronomical satellite, sent into space in 1981, has discovered over 200,000 objects previously unknown to humans. What is this satellite called?

Quazar   Ethel

Probe 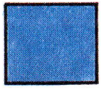   Iris

Venus is the brightest planet in our solar system. It is so bright it can sometimes be seen with the naked eye during the day. What makes Venus appear so bright?

Volcanic eruptions 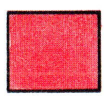   Surface clouds

Vast deserts    Large oceans

The first 50 miles of the earth's atmosphere is made up of 78 percent nitrogen, 21 percent oxygen and small amounts of argon, carbon dioxide and other gases. How thick is the earth's total atmosphere?

400 miles    1,500 feet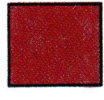

35 miles    120 miles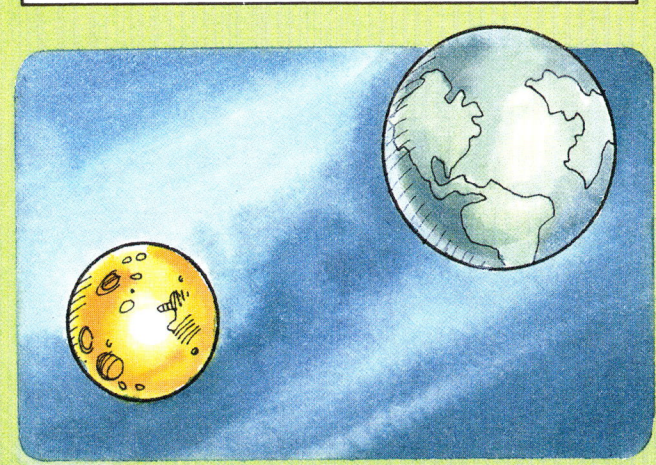

CAN YOU COMPUTE?

The first commercial computers were huge pieces of equipment that occupied whole rooms. By comparison, today's computers are minute, but they have a much greater capacity to store information and perform calculations.

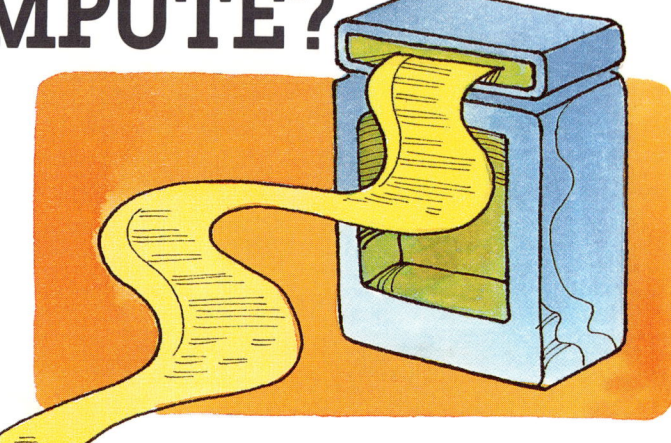

Read each question. Then press **QUESTRON** on the colored square next to the right answer.

The most commonly used computers are called digital computers. What is a digit?

A unit of electricity	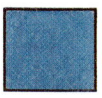	A memory cell	
A number		A split second	

A digital watch contains a microchip that can show the time, give alarm signals, do calculations and even play tunes. What vital mineral is necessary to make a digital watch work?

Mercury		Zinc	
Diamonds		Quartz	

Scientists have used computers to design microprocessors. These are tiny chips that hold thousands of storage units and can be programmed to control other machines. What are the chips made of?

Rhodium	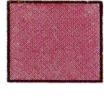	Copper	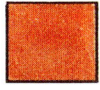
Silicon		Silver	

Computers could not have been developed without the invention of the transistor, an electronic device used to amplify electrical currents. When was the transistor invented?

1948	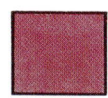	1912	
1966	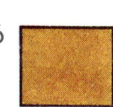	1939	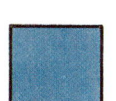

Today's "supercomputers" are able to perform over 100 million arithmetic operations each second. The first fully electronic digital computer was completed in 1946. How many operations per second was it able to perform?

5,000		500,000	
550		5,000,000	

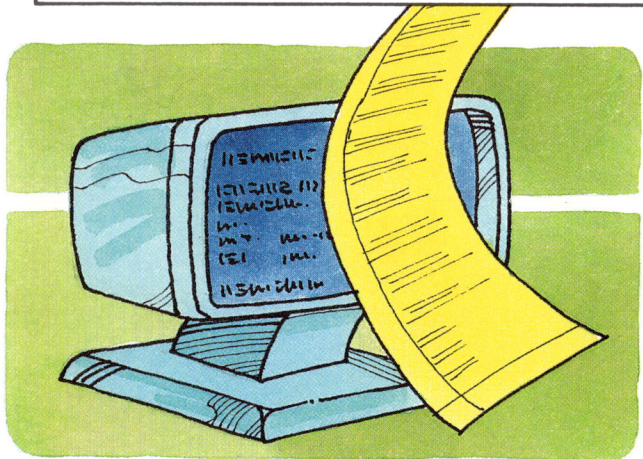

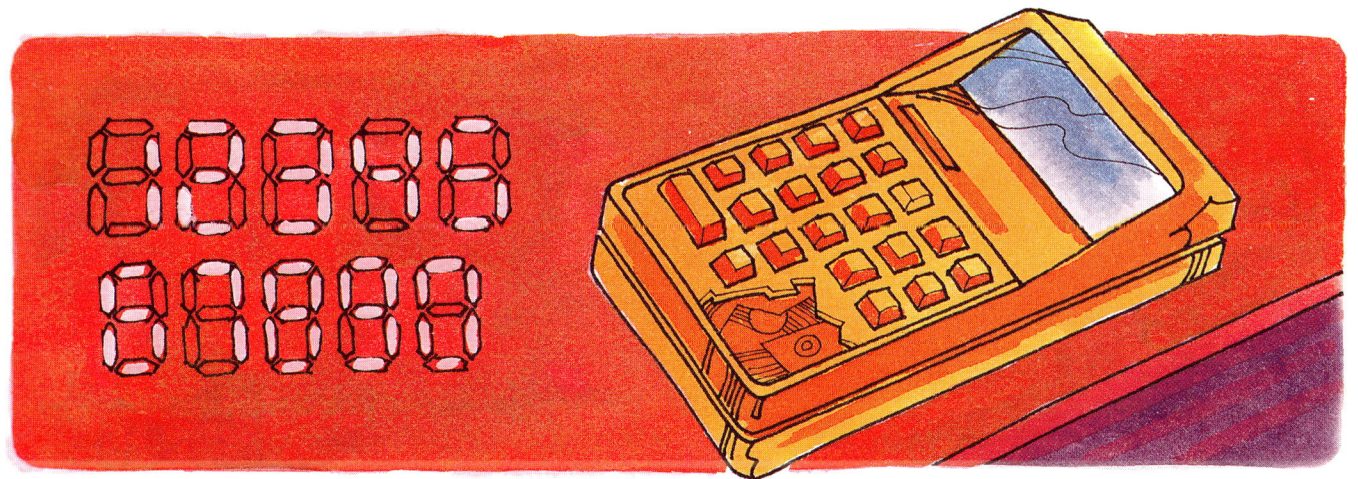

Digital computers use the binary number system. The binary system uses just two units, 0 and 1, unlike the decimal system, which uses 10 units. What are the binary units called?

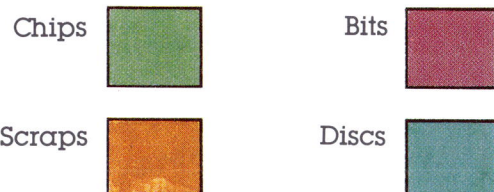

- Chips
- Bits
- Scraps
- Discs

Tiny electronic calculators can work out complicated mathematical problems at speeds equivalent to the speed of light. How fast is that?

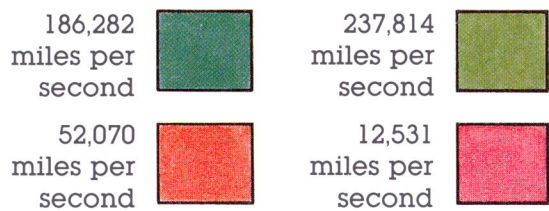

- 186,282 miles per second
- 237,814 miles per second
- 52,070 miles per second
- 12,531 miles per second

Thousands of companies worldwide produce computer hardware and software. The hardware is the actual computer, and includes the electronic and magnetic devices. What does "software" normally refer to?

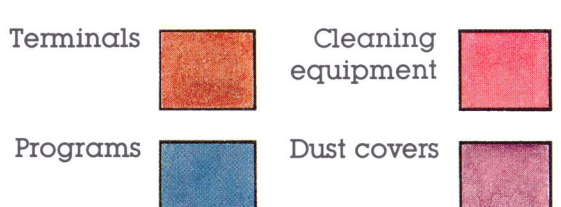

- Terminals
- Cleaning equipment
- Programs
- Dust covers

Computers can be linked to high speed communication lines that allow operators located many miles apart to work on a single program at the same time. What is this system known as?

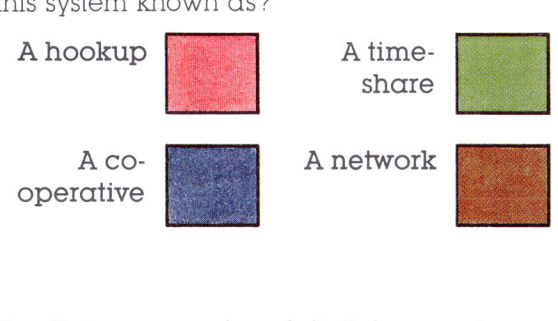

- A hookup
- A time-share
- A co-operative
- A network

The first mass-produced digital computer was introduced in 1951. It was called UNIVAC 1 (**UNIV**ersal **A**utomatic **C**omputer). Who do you think ordered the first one?

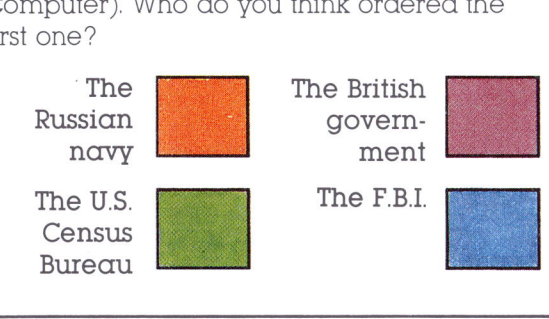

- The Russian navy
- The British government
- The U.S. Census Bureau
- The F.B.I.

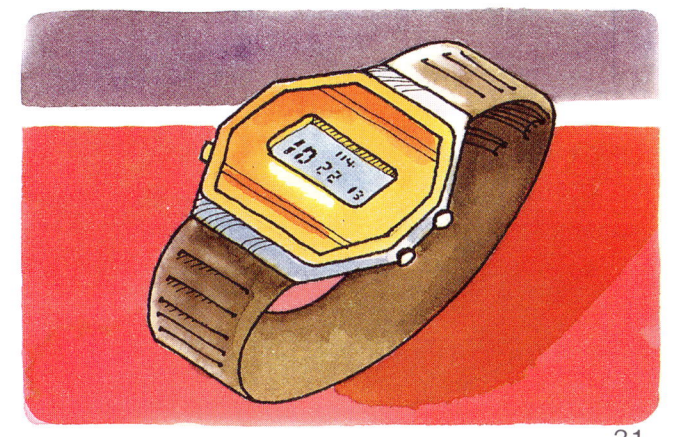

THE QUESTRON™ LIBRARY OF ELECTRONIC BOOKS

A series of books specially designed to
reach—and teach—and entertain children of all ages

QUESTRON ELECTRONIC WORKBOOKS

Early Childhood

My First Counting Book
My First ABC Book
My First Book of Animals
Shapes and Sizes
Pre-School Skills
My First Vocabulary
My First Nursery Rhymes
Autos, Ships, Trains and Planes
Reading Readiness
My First Words
My First Numbers
Going Places
Kindergarten Skills

Grades 1-5

My First Reading Book *(K-1)*
First Grade Skills *(1)*
My First Book of Addition *(1-2)*
My First Book of Multiplication *(2-3)*
I Want to Be... *(2-5)*
Number Fun *(2-5)*
Word Fun *(2-5)*

ELECTRONIC QUIZBOOKS FOR THE WHOLE FAMILY

Trivia Fun and Games	More, How, Why, Where and When
How, Why, Where and When	World Records and Amazing Facts

PRICE/STERN/SLOAN — **RANDOM HOUSE, INC.**
Publishers, Inc., Los Angeles   *New York*